2013

Oakes'

Clinical Practitioner's
Pocket Guide
To

Respiratory
Care

D1237024

Dana F. Oakes
Scot N. Jones

RespiratoryBooks

a division of:
Health Educator Publications, Inc.
10690 NW 6th St
Coral Springs, FL 33071

AUTHORS

Dana F. Oakes, BA, RRT-NPS

Educational Consultant

Formerly:
Director of Respiratory Care
VA Medical Center
Washington, D.C.

Educational Coordinator/Instructor
Respiratory Care Department
Children's Hospital National Medical Center
Washington, D.C.

Director of Clinical Education
Respiratory Care Program
Columbia Union College
Tacoma Park, MD, USA

Scot N. Jones, BA, RRT, RCP

Director of Clinical Education

Broward College
Coconut Creek, FL

ISBN 978-0-932887-42-9

RespiratoryBooks
A Division of Health Educator Publications, Inc.
10690 NW 6th St
Coral Springs, FL 33071

Table of Contents
(at-a-glance)

2013 – Eighth Edition

**Turn to Page 1 of each chapter for a
DETAILED TABLE OF CONTENTS**

Important Disclaimer:

Preface

It is difficult to believe that the "Blue Book" is quickly approaching its 30th Birthday, having now entered the 8th edition. It has been a tremendous collective effort over the years, for which we are deeply appreciative of the support and feedback we've received.

The book is also a reflection of the progression of where we've come from, from transporting gases throughout the hospital corridors to today's invaluable physician-extenders. The book has grown into a whole group of books. Each edition is a fight between adding what is new and relevant with trading out what belongs in more specialized titles. These are indeed exciting times.

If you haven't experienced it, we also invite you to check out our newest addition to the family: RespiratoryUpdate.com. RespiratoryUpdate combines searchable, full text all of the Oakes' Pocket Guides with hundreds of hand-picked web resources, internationally moderated expert forums, and more!

Thank you for joining us on the journey. Keep pushing us forward!

Acknowledgements

Always first and foremost, we are thankful for our Lord, Jesus Christ, for His allowing us to play this small part in our field. To Him, and to Him only goes the Glory.

We also humbly acknowledge the incredible efforts of all the Assistant Editors whom have created an incredible edition.

1 PATIENT ASSESSMENT

CONTENTS

Health History	
Obtain the following (do not limit to pulmonary):	
Demographics	Including name, address, gender, age, place of birth, nationality, marital status, occupation, religion and race. NOTE source of history (and reliability), overall condition, and Chief Complaint (CC).
Past Medical	Including childhood diseases, all significant illnesses/injuries, and hospitalizations. Include those untreated.
Family	Four generations of all illnesses/diseases
Social	Hobbies, recreation, living arrangements, social activities, habits, substance abuse, and travel.
Emotional	Satisfaction with life, stress, relationships, finances, Psychiatric illnesses

(Continued Next Page)

Occupational Environmental	**Work or Live Around:** Farms, Foundries, Mills, Mines, Shipyards, Asbestos, Dust, Fumes, Gases, Smoke, Toxic Chemicals, etc. **Home Irritants:** Air conditioning, Glue, Humidifiers, Insulation, Paint, Pets, Smoking, Woodpiles, Mold **Geographic fungi (region)** See Ch 11: Histoplasmosis, Asbestosis, Aspergillis, etc.
Cardio-pulmonary **Smoking Hx:** *Pack Years =* (# Yrs Smoked) X (# Packs/Day)	**Pulmonary:** Allergies, Asthma, Bronchiectasis, Bronchitis, CA, Colds, CF, Fungal Infections, Influenza, Lupus, PNA, Pneumothorax, Pleurisy, Sinus Infections, Sleep Apneas, Alpha-1, etc. **Cardiovascular:** CHD, Diabetes, MI, Heart Failure, HTN, Obesity, Surgery, Trauma **Drug Abuse:** There is often a correlation between respiratory problems and illicit drug abuse. Encourage honesty **Habits:** Alcohol, Caffeine, Diet, Exercise, Sleep
Review of Systems	A list of questions looking at body systems to uncover problems related to Chief Complaint (CC)
History of Present Illness (HPI)	Chron. description of: Each Symptom (see pg 1-15); Onset; Location (Radiating?); Timing (Freq, Duration); Character (Quality, Quantity, Severity)
Cardio Care/ Medications	Current Cardiopulmonary Care and Medications (including OTC)
Review of Physician's Orders	

Respectful Bedside Assessment

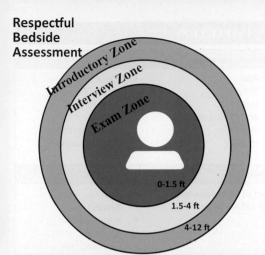

Introductory Zone

Interview Zone

Exam Zone

0-1.5 ft

1.5-4 ft

4-12 ft

Introduction (establish a positive rapport, obtain patient's cooperation, determine overall patient condition, assess environment for safety)
- Address pt. by formal name - avoid extremes in friendliness
- Introduce Yourself; Explain your professional role and state purpose of visit
- Be warm, friendly, and professional (clean, neat, eye contact)

Interview (obtain information concerning CC and further develop positive rapport)
- Provide necessary privacy
- Use appropriate eye contact, and avoid standing at foot of bed
- Maintain a relaxed style; be honest; communicate empathy
- Never argue or make moral judgments
- Use Interpreter if needed, use non-medical language (no jargon)

Physical Exam (determine condition of patient and insure prescribed treatment is appropriate)
- Request permission to check ID and to perform exam
- Use minimal/no eye contact, only necessary touch, min. verbal
- Be aware of patient's response
- Use appropriate PPE to establish professional/infectious barriers

INSPECTION

General Appearance

- Age
- Weight
- Height
- Body Structure
- Skin Color
- Hygiene
- Culture
- Level of Distress
- Motor Activity
- Nutrition
- Physical limitations
- Sensory limitations

Mental Status

Level of Consciousness
(see details on pg 1-21)

- Anxiety
- Restlessness
- Altered Speech
- Confusion
- Disorientation

Cardiopulmonary Distress

Anxiety
- Cool Hands
- Sweaty Palms
- Fidgety
- Restless
- Tense

Body Position
- Leaning on elbows?

Chest Pain
- Guarding
- Moaning
- Shallow Breaths
- Writhing

Breathing
- Choking
- Gurgling
- Coughing
- Dyspnea
- Irregular Pattern
- Labored
- Rapid
- Shallow
- Wheezing

see pg 1-11 for breathing patterns

Personality and Attitude

- Responses towards their illness
- Responses towards you
- Resistive
- Crossed Arms
- Lack of Eye Contact
- Brief, Curt Responses

Vital Signs: Normal and Abnormal Ranges

See Oakes' Hemodynamic Monitoring for detailed instructions on Pulse and BP monitoring

Age	Respiratory Rate	Heart Rate	Blood Pressure
Adult	12-16	60-100	110-120/70-80
5-12 yrs	16-20	70-110	100/60
1-4 yrs	20-30	80-120	95/50
1st year	25-40	80-160	85/50
Newborn	30-50	90-180	75/40
Adult Abnormal ranges	< 12 = bradypnea > 20 = tachypnea	< 60 = bradycardia > 100 = tachycardia	< 90/60 = hypotension > 140/90 = hypertension
Notes	See page 1-11 for respiratory patterns	Pulse deficit = difference between auscultated beats and peripheral pulse Check equality of pulse strengths in all major arteries: Right vs. Left Upper vs. Lower extremities Inspiration vs. Expiration	Mean BP = BPsys + 2 BPdia / 3 (adult normal = 93) Pulse Pressure (PP) = BPsys - BPdia (adult normal = 40)

Strength (amplitude) of Pulse

4 - bounding	1 - diminished
3 - full, increased	0 - absent
2 - normal	

Heart Rhythms

Pulsus Alternans	Regular alteration of weak and strong pulses
Pulsus Corrigans	Strong or Bounding, with ↑PP
Pulsus Parvus	Weak Pulse with ↓PP
Pulsus Paradoxus	↓ Pulse Strength during Inspiration; ↑ during Expiration (> 10 mmHg is signif., > 20 is needed to feel the difference)
Reverse Pulsus Paradoxus	Reverse of above - as noted during Positive Pressure Ventilation

Pulse Oximetry (SpO2)

	Normal	Hypoxemia		
		Mild	Moderate	Severe
Adult	95-99%	91-94%	76-90%	< 75%
Child	91-96%	88-90%	76-87%	< 75%

Pulse Oximetry Quick Troubleshooting	
Check:	• Good Perfusion? • Good Waveform? • Skin Temperature at Probe? • Ambient Light or Nailpolish?
Try:	• Switch position or type of probe • Replace probe • Cover Probe (if bright room) • Warm body part with approved heat pack • Verify using ABG if necessary

Temperature

Core (Most Accurate)	Intermediate (Affected by Body, Environment)
• Pulmonary Artery • Esophageal Probe • Nasopharynx • Tympanic (Ear) • Jugular Bulb	• Sublingual (under tongue) • Axillary (under arm) • Rectal • Forehead • Bladder

Normal Temperature Ranges

Place	Celsius Range	Fahrenheit Range
Core	36.5 – 37.5° C	97.7 – 99.5° F
Oral*	36.5 – 37.5° C	97.7 – 99.5° F
Axillary	35.9 – 36.9° C	96.7 – 98.5° F
Otic (tympanic)	37.1 – 38.1° C	98.7 – 100.5° F

*Cool or heated aerosol may affect temperature readings

Causes of Abnormal Temperatures
(defined as those outside of the above Normal Temp Ranges)

Hypothermia	Hyperthermia (rapid onset, diffic. to control, doesn't respond to antipyretics)
• Environmental Exposure • Extremes of Age • Brain/Spinal Injuries • Shock • Anesthesia • Sedation • Therapeutic (MI)	• Environmental Exposure • Malignant (Drug-Related) • Brain/Spinal Injuries
	Fever (usually responds to antipyretics)
	• Infection (w/ ↑ WBC)

Thoracic Cage Landmarks

ANTERIOR

Top of lungs
(2-4 cm above
middle of clavicles)

Suprasternal notch
(top of manubrium)

Sternal angle
(angle of Louis)
(articulation of 2nd rib
and bifurcation of
trachea)

Xiphoid Process

Costal Angles

Bottom of lungs
6th rib midclavicular
8th rib midaxillary
(at end exhal.)

Costal margins

POSTERIOR

C-7 -- most prominent
spinous process at base
of neck

T-1 -- next spinous
process below C-7,
articulation of 1st rib and
top of lungs

T-4 -- tracheal bifurcation

T-8 -- inferior angle of
scapulae

T-9 -- top of right dome
of diaphragm and bottom
of right lung (at end exp.)

T-10 -- top of left dome
of diaphragm and bottom
of left lung (at end
expiration

**Chest Topography
Imaginary Lines**

Front:
mid-sternal
R + L midclavicular

Side:
anterior axillary
midaxillary
posterior axillary

Back:
midspinal (vertebral)
midscapular

1-8

Topographic Position of the Lungs and Heart

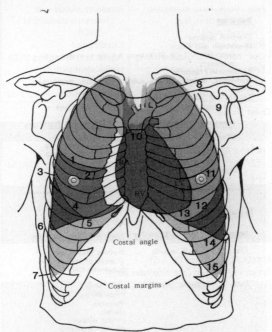

1. Transverse fissure
2. 4th rib midclavicular
3. Oblique fissure at 5th rib midaxillary
4. Oblique fissure
5. Lung border during expiration(6th rib midclav)
6. Lung border during expiration(8th rib mid axill)
7. Pleural border (10th rib midaxillary)
8. Clavicle
9. Scapula
10. Aorta
11. Nipple (4th intercostal space in male)
12. Oblique fissure
13. Apex of heart (PMI at 5th intercostal space)
14. Lung border during expiration(8th rib midaxillary)
15. Pleural border (10th rib midaxillary)

1-9

Head and Neck

Head	Neck
Face: Color, facial expression (alert, distress, fear, mood, pain) **Nose**: Nasal flaring **Lips**: Color, pursed lip breathing **Eyes**: Pupillary reflexes Mydriasis = fixed & dilate Miosis = pinpoint	**Accessory muscle use** ($\uparrow$sternocleidomastoid = $\uparrow$WOB) **Carotid pulse** **Jugular vein distention** (JVD) **Lymphadenopathy** (infection, HIV) **Tracheal position** see pg 1-12

Chest Shape

Diameter	Rib Angles	Symmetry
Normal AP diameter = 1/2 to 2/3 (> 2/3 = barrel chest)	Normal = 45° COPD = horizontal	Flail chest Pneumothorax Splinting

Deformities:
Lesions, obesity, muscular atrophy/hypertrophy, rib fractures, scars, spine (kyphosis, scoliosis), sternum (pectus carinatum/excavatum)

Breathing Rate (see Pg. 1-5)
Breathing Pattern (see also next page)

I/E Ratio Posture SOB (dyspnea while talking, nasal flaring, pursed-lip) Orthopnea = SOB lying down Platypnea = SOB upright Accessory muscle use: substernal, suprasternal, intercostal, bulging, retractions, clavicular lift, splinting Symmetry – uni or bilateral	Abdominal distension (ascites, obesity, pregnancy) Excursion (depth): Chest vs. abdomen Respiratory alternans–chest wall breathing alternating with diaphragm breathing Paradoxical (flail chest) Abdominal paradox (abdomen inward during inspiration)

Restriction: Typically rapid/shallow breathing
Obstruction: Typically $\uparrow T_E$ = lower airway; $\uparrow T_I$ = upper airway
Paroxysmal Nocturnal Dyspnea (PND) = SOB and coughing (generally at night)

Breathing Patterns

Type	Pattern	Characteristics	Causes
Eupnea		Normal rate (12 - 20 bpm) Normal rhythm, Sighs 7/hr	Normal physiology
Apnea		Absence of breathing	Respiratory or cardiac arrest, ↑ICP
Bradypnea		Slow rate (< 10 bpm), regular rhythm	Normal during sleep, brain tumors, diabetic coma, drugs (alcohol, narcotics), ↑ICP, metabolic alkalosis (limited), uremia
Tachypnea		↑ Rate (> 25 bpm), regular rhythm	Anxiety (esp. asthmatics), atelectasis, brain lesions, drugs (aspirin), exercise, fear, fever, hypercapnia, hypoxemia, hypoxia, metabolic acidosis, obesity, pain
Hypopnea		↓ Depth, normal rate, regular rhythm	Circulatory failure, meningitis, unconsciousness
Hyperpnea		↑ Depth, normal rate, regular rhythm	Exertion, fever, pain, respiratory disease
Apneustic		Long gasping inspirations with insufficient expiration	Lesions in the pneumotaxic center
Biot's		Fast and deep breaths with periods of apnea, no set rhythm	Spinal meningitis, ↑ICP, CNS lesions or disease
Cheynes-Stokes		↑ Breaths (rate & depth) then decreasing breaths followed by periods of apnea (20-60 sec)	Normal in newborns and aged, CHF, aortic valve lesion, dissecting aneurysm, ↑ICP, ↑CO2 sensitivity meningitis, cerebral anoxia, drug overdose (morphine), renal failure
Kussmaul's		Fast and deep breaths like sighs with no expiratory phase	DKA, severe hemorrhage, peritonitis, renal failure, uremia

1-11

PALPATION

Tracheal Position	Chest & Diaphragm Excursion
(shift from midline) **Shift towards**: unilateral upper lobe collapse **Shift away**: lung tumor, pleural effusion, tension pneumothorax	**Normal**: 3 cm women, 4-6 cm men (posteriorly) **Unilateral ↓** : atlectasis, lobar consolidation, pleural effusion, pneumothorax **Bilateral ↓** : COPD, NM disease

Tactile (vocal) fremitus	Skin - bruises, masses,
feeling vocal vibrations when patient says "99" with a low-pitched voice	subcutaneous emphysema, turgor **PMI, Tenderness, fractures**

↓Fremitus Vibrations	↑Fremitus Vibrations
Airflow↓: Obstruction (COPD, secretions), restriction (shallow breathing), ET tube malposition **Barrier**: Air – COPD, pneumothorax Fat – Obesity Fibrosis – Pleural thickening Fluid – Pleural effusion Muscle – Hypertrophy	**Consolidation**: Atelectasis Fibrosis Infarct Pneumonia Tumor

PERCUSSION

Note	Normal Areas	Abnormal Areas
Flat	Thigh, muscle	Massive atelectasis or pleural effusion, pneumonectomy
Dull	Heart, liver	Atelectasis, consolid., enlarged heart, fibrosis, neoplasm, pleural effusion or thicken., pulm. edema
Resonance	Normal lung	
Hyperreso-nance	Abdomen	Acute asthma, emphysema, pneumothorax
Tympany	Large gastric air bubble	Large pulmonary cavity, tension pneumothorax

AUSCULTATION

Normal Breath Sounds

Type	Description	I:E
Vesicular	Normal sound over most of lungs	3:1 breezy
Bronchovesicular	Normal sound over carina area and between upper scapulae	1:1 breezy/tubular
Bronchial	Normal sound over manubrium	2:3 hollow/tubular/loud
Tracheal	Normal sound over upper trachea	5:6 tubular/loud/harsh

Abnormal Breath Sounds(see also Adventitious, next page)

↓Breath Sounds	↑Breath Sounds
Airflow ↓: Obstruction (COPD, secretions), restriction (shallow breathing), ET tube malpos. **Barrier:** Air – COPD, pneumothorax Fat – Obesity Fibrosis – Pleural thickening; Fluid – Pleural effusion Muscle – Hypertrophy	**Consolidation:** Atelectasis Fibrosis Infarct Pneumonia Tumor

Voice Sounds (Vocal Resonance)

Type	Normal	Abnormal
Bronchophony	Spoken syllables are non-distinct	↑ distinction = consolidation
Whispered pectoriloquy	Whispers are faint & non-distinct	↓ distinction = air or fluid insulation
Egophony	Spoken E → E	Spoken E→ A = lung consolid over a pleural effusion

Distinguishing Between Air, Solid (consolidation), and Fluid (pleural) in the Chest Cavity

		↑ Presence of:		
Method	Sign	Air	Solid	Fluid
Palpation	Fremitus	↓	↑	↓
Percussion	Resonance	↑	↓	↓
Auscultation	Breath sounds	↓	↑	↓

1-13

Adventitious Breath Sounds *

Type	Description	Probable Location	Common Causes
Crackle – Discontinuous vibrations	*Fine* – High pitched crackling at end inspiration *Medium* – Wetter and louder at any part of inspiration *Coarse* – Loud, low-pitched bubbling at expiration or inspir.	*Alveoli* – Atelectasis or excessive fluid *Bronchioles* – Air moving through fluid *Larger airways* – Air moving through fluid, may clear w/ cough	Atelectasis, fibrosis, pneumonia, pulmonary edema Bronchitis, emphysema, pneumonia, pulmonary edema Bronchitis, emphysema, pneumonia, pulmonary edema
Wheeze – Continuous vibrations	Musical – usually occurs during expiration, but may occur during inspiration	*High pitch:* Lower airway squeak due to narrowing *Low pitch* (rhonchi): Upper airway snore (usually due to sputum production that may disappear with cough)	Asthma, bronchitis, CHF, emphysema, foreign body, mucous plug, stenosis, tumor
Stridor – Continuous vibrations	Loud, high-pitched crowing in upper airway, usually during inspiration	Usually due to upper airway obstruction (usually inspir = above glottis; expir = lower trachea)	Croup, epiglottitis, foreign body, tracheal stenosis, tumor, vocal cord edema
Rub – Pleural or pericardial	Grating vibration, loud & harsh *Pleural:* Assoc. with I & E *Pericardial:* Assoc. with heart beat	*Pleural* – pleural membrane rub *Pericardial* – pericardial sac rub	Pleurisy, peripheral pneumonia, pulmonary emboli, TB Pericarditis

* As recommended by ACCP-ATS Joint Committee on Pulmonary Nomenclature, 1975 and updates

1-14

OTHER RESPIRATORY ASSESSMENTS

Fingers	Tremors, Yellow Stains, Clubbing (see Ch 11)
Sputum	See Ch 5
Skin and Mucous Membranes	
Capillary Refill	Color return to fingernail within 3 sec, after a 5 sec pinch. > 3 sec = ↓CO or poor digital perfusion.
Temperature	Cold (cool room, ↓ circulation) Warm/flushed (warm room, anxiety, embarassment, fever, hypercapnia)
Rashes, bruises, lesions	Note age of bruising, lesions. Ask about Rashes - New? Medication related?
Color	Pallor, Flush, Cyanosis
Peripheral	(acrocyanosis) - Poor Circulation
Central Cyanosis	Poor Bld Oxygenat.
Edema	Legs, Ankles

Pitting Scale	
1+	rapid
2+	10-15 seconds
3+	1-2 minutes
4+	> 2 minutes

Pulmonary Symptoms: General questions to Consider

1. Cough:
sound, productive?, frequency and duration, onset, triggers, severity

2. Dyspnea:
Inspiratory (Upper Airway) vs. Expiratory (Lower Airways), PND, Orthopnea, Platypnea, frequency and duration, onset, triggers, severity

3. Chest Pain:
Pleuritic or not?, frequency and duration, location and radiation, triggers, severity

4. Hemoptysis:
amount, odor, frequency and duration, severity (massive = 300 mL in 3 hrs or 600 mL in 24 hours) (See also Chapter 5)

Common Disease Assessment Findings

Disease	Inspection	Palpation	Percussion	Auscultation
Asthma	↑RR, ↑TE, dyspnea, ↑accessory muscle use, nasal flaring, orthopnea, ↑A-P diameter	Normal or ↓ fremitus	Normal or hyper resonance (?)	↓BS (severe ↓ = danger), wheezes, crackles, ↑TE
Atelectasis	↑RR, dyspnea, ↓ chest expansion (same side), cyanosis (?), tracheal deviation (same side)	↑ fremitus	Dull	↑ or ↓BS, crackles (fine), whispered pectoriloquy
Chronic Bronchitis	↑RR, ↑TE, dyspnea, ↑accessory muscle use, fat or stocky, ↑A-P diameter, chronic cough, cyanosis, ↓ diaphragm movement	Normal or ↓ fremitus	Normal to dull	↓BS, crackles (all types), wheeze
Emphysema	↑RR, ↑TE, dyspnea, orthopnea, pursed-lip breathing, hypertrophy of accessory muscles, thin, ↑A-P diameter, ↓ chest movement, ↓ diaphragm movement	Normal or ↓ fremitus	Hyper-resonance	↓BS, crackles (all types), wheeze
Large mass	Usually normal	↓ fremitus (AW occluded) ↑ fremitus (if not)	Dull	↓BS (if airway occluded) ↑Bronchial BS (if not) Crackles (fine), rub (maybe)
Pleural effusion	↑ RR, dyspnea, ↓ chest movement (same side), tracheal deviation (opposite side), cyanosis	↓ fremitus	Dull or flat (may be only way to distinguish from a pneumothorax)	↓BS, pleural rub (maybe), egophony (above effusion)

1-16

Disease	Inspection	Palpation	Percussion	Auscultation
Pleural thickening	↓ chest movement (same side),	↓ fremitus	Dull	↓BS
Pneumonia	↑RR, dyspnea, cough, ↓ chest movement (same side), pleuritic pain (maybe), cyanosis (maybe), fever	↑ fremitus	Dull	↓BS +/or ↑ bronchial BS, crackles (vary with stage), pleural rub (maybe), bronchophony
Pneumo-thorax	↑RR, dyspnea, ↓ chest movement and expanded if closed, tracheal deviation (same side, other side if tension), cyanosis	↓ fremitus	Hyper-resonance or tympany	↓BS
Pulmonary edema	↑RR, dyspnea, orthopnea, ↑accessory muscle use, pale or cyanosis	↑ fremitus	Dull	↑ bronchovesicular BS, crackles (medium), wheeze (maybe)
Pulmonary embolism	↑RR, dyspnea, ↑HR, apprehension, cough, sharp chest pain, hemoptysis	Normal	Normal	↓BS (locally), crackles, wheeze, pleural rub (locally)
Pulmonary interstitial fibrosis	Rapid, shallow breathing, ↑accessory muscle use, dyspnea on exertion, cyanosis (late), clubbing (maybe)	Normal or ↑ fremitus	Normal or dull	↑ bronchovesicular BS (maybe), crackles (fine), whispered pectoriloquy

1-17

Assessment of Oxygenation (See Chapter 10)

Assessment of Ventilation:

	Norm.	Ab-norm		Norm.	Ab-norm
Adequacy			**Efficiency**		
$\dot{V}_E$	5-7 L/min	↑↓	V_D phys	$1/3\dot{V}_E$	↑↓
$PaCO_2$	35-45mmHg	↑↓	V_D/V_T	0.33-0.45	↑↓
$P_{ET}CO_2$	35-43 mmHg (4.6 - 5.6%)	↑↓			
$Pa_{-ET}CO_2$	1-5 mmHg	> 6 mmHg			

Assessment of Load (ventilatory mechanics)

Adequacy	Normal	Abnormal
Cdyn	40-70 mL/cm H_2O	↓
Cstat	70-100 mL/cm H_2O	↓
Raw	0.5 - 2.5 cm H_2O / L / sec @ 0.5 L / sec (4-8 with ET tube)	> 15 cmH2O/L/sec
RSBI (f/VT)	<105	>105

Assessment of Capacity (ventilatory mechanics)

	Normal	Abnormal
Adequacy		
Respiratory Drive (P0.1)	< 2 cm H_2O	> 4-6 cm H_2O
Resp. Muscle Strength		
VC	60-80 mL/kg	< 60 mL/kg
PImax (MIP, NIF)	< -60 cm H_2O	> -30 cmH2O
Resp. Muscle Endurance		
MVV	120-180 L/min	< 20 L/min
$\dot{V}_E$/MVV	< 1:2	> 1:2

CARDIOVASCULAR ASSESSMENT

Heart

Inspection/Palpation

PMI-5th left IC space, mid-clavicular line; often ↓ in COPD and shifted down to left sternal border; shifts towards a lobar collapse and away from a tension pneumothorax; shifts left in cardiomegaly

Pulmonic Area - 2nd left IC space near sternal border, ↑ vibrations with pulmonary hypertension

> **Pulse and BP monitoring** - See Oakes' Hemodynamic Monitoring for detailed instructions

Auscultation - Heart sounds

S1	S2
Closure of A-V valves (ventricular contraction), beginning systole, loudest at apex.	Closure of semilunar valves (ventricular relaxation), during diastole, loudest at base. Split may be normal (↑ during I) Split abnormal (width ↑) in pulmonary hypertension or stenosis.

S3	S4
Rapid ventricular filling during diastole, abnormal except in young, healthy children. Associated with CHF	Active filling of ventricles by atrial contraction (late diastole), may be normal and abnormal

Intensity

Normal = clear sounds	**Abnormal** ↑ = pulmonary hypertension (S2), cor pulmonale
At base of heart: S1 < S2	**Abnormal** ↓ (distant or muffled) =
At apex of heart: S1 > S2	heart failure, obesity, pneumothorax, pulm hyperinflation, valve abnorm.

Abnormal Heart Sounds

Gallop Rhythms	Murmurs	
Ventricular gallop: Abnormal presence of S3 **Atrial gallop:** Abnormal presence of S4	I Barely audible II Audible III Moderately loud IV Loud, no thrill V Very loud, thrill VI Audible off chest	**Systolic:** Incompetent AV or stenotic semilunar **Diastolic:** Incompetent semilunar or stenotic AV

1-19

FLUID & ELECTROLYTE ASSESSMENT

Urine Output:

Average	1,200 mL / Day	~40 mL / hr
Male	900-1,800 mL/Day	or > 0.5 mL/kg/hr
Female	600-1,600 mL/Day	

Normal Electrolyte Values affecting Ventil. Muscles:

Potassium	K^+	3.5-5.0 mEq/L
Magnesium	Mg^{++}	1.3-2.5 mEq/L
Phosphate	$PO^{4=}$	1.4-2.7 mEq/L

Fluid Balance Assessment

Fluid Excess	Fluid Deficit
↑body weight, ↑CO, ↑BP	↓body weight, ↓BP(postural)
↑PAP, ↑CVP , ↑JVD	↑HR, ↓PAP, ↓CVP, ↓JVD
↓Hgb, ↓Hct	↑Hgb,↑Hct
Bounding pulse	Poor peripheral pulse
Moist mucous membranes	Dry mucous membranes
Pitting edema	Extremities: cool/pale &
Pulmonary edema	trunk: warm/dry, ↓skin
↑UO from overload	elasticity
↓UO (< 0.5 mL/kg/hr x 2 hr)	↑UO (diuresis)
	↓ capillary refill

Changes in Fluid Balance - Causes of

↑Fluid (Hypervolemia)		↓Fluid (Hypovolemia)	
↑Intake	↓Output	↓Intake	↑Output
Iatrogenic	↓**Renal Perfusion:**	Dehydration	Burns
	Heart Failure	Starvation	Diarrhea
	PPV (↓CO, ↑ADH)		Diuresis
	Renal System	**Fluid Shift:**	Hemorrhage
	Malfunction	Burns, Shock	Vomiting
	Blocked Foley		

NEUROLOGICAL ASSESSMENT

Vital Signs	RR, HR, BP
Motor Activity	Ability to cough/clear secretions
	Grip strength
	Motions: coordination, paralysis, tremors
	Posture:
	Decorticate – flexed arms, extended legs,
	plantar flexion
	Decerebrate- extended arms, extended legs,
	plantar flexion
	Pupil size and reaction
Mental Status	Emotional state, behavior, comfort, orientation
	LOC – See below

15
Fully Alert
↓
3
Comatose

EYES OPEN	
Spontaneously	4
To speech	3
To pain	2
Not at all	1

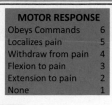

MOTOR RESPONSE	
Obeys Commands	6
Localizes pain	5
Withdraw from pain	4
Flexion to pain	3
Extension to pain	2
None	1

VERBAL RESPONSE	
Oriented	5
Confused	4
Inappropriate	3
Incomprehensible	2
None	1

MODIFIED GLASGOW COMA SCORE

Minor ≥ 13
Moderate 9-12
Severe ≤ 8

See Oakes' Neonatal/Pediatric Respiratory Care for Other Resources

Descriptive Terms for Level of Consciousness (LOC)

Alert:	Awake, oriented and responds appropriately
Confusion:	Inability to think clearly, impaired judgment
Disorientation:	Starting loss of consc., disoriented to time/place
Lethargic:	Sleepy, arouses easily, responds appropriately
Obtunded:	Awakens only with diff.; then responds appropriately
Stuporous:	Does not completely awaken, responds only to deep pain, withdraws or pushes you away
Unresponsive:	Responds only to deep pain, exhibits reflex
Comatose:	No response, flaccid muscle tone

2 ARTERIAL BLOOD GASES

Oxygenation Aspects of ABG's are Covered in Chapter 10: Respiratory Procedures

► Indicates AARC Clinical Practice Guideline

Normal ABG Parameters		Mixed Venous	
	Range	Norm	Range
pH (pHa, pH$\bar{v}$), units	7.35-7.45	7.36	7.31-7.41
PCO$_2$ (PaCO$_2$, P$\bar{V}$CO$_2$), mmHg	35-45	46	41-51
PO$_2$ (PaO$_2$, P$\bar{V}$O$_2$), mmHg*	80-100	40	35-42
O$_2$ Sat (SaO$_2$, S$\bar{V}$O$_2$), %	95-100%	75%	68-77%
HCO$_3$, mEq/L	22-26	24	22-26
TCO$_2$	23-27	25	23-27
BE, mEq/L	+/- 2	0	+/- 2
O$_2$ content (CaO$_2$, C$\bar{V}$O$_2$), mL/dL	15-24	15	12-15

*21% O$_2$ at sea level

Sampling for Arterial Blood Gas Analysis[1, 2]
(AARC CPG)

Indications

Need to evaluate:
Oxygenation (PaO$_2$, SaO$_2$, HbO$_2$, Hgb total, dyshemoglobins)
Ventilation (PaCO$_2$)
Acid-base (pH, PaCO$_2$)
Need to quantitate patient's response to: therapy and/or diagnostic evaluation.
Monitor disease severity and progression.

Contraindications

Hand puncture – negative Allen test
Any limb site – infection, PVD, surgical shunt
Femoral puncture –outside the hospital
Coagulopathy or anticoagulant therapy (relative)

Hazards/Complications

Anaphlaxis (local anesthetic)
Arterial occlusion
Arteriospasm
Contagion at site
Emboli (air or blood)
Hematoma
Hemorrhage
Pain
Trauma to vessel
Vagovagal response

Monitoring

Patient: RR, temperature, clinical appearance, position and/or activity level, puncture site (post sample).
O$_2$/vent therapy: proper application of O$_2$ device , FIO$_2$ or flowrate, ventilator mode and settings.
Procedure: ease or difficulty, pulsatile blood return, air bubbles or clot.

Frequency

Dependent on clinical status and indication, alternate sites or A-line is indicated for multiple sampling.

Clinical Goals

(desired outcome)
Sample obtained without contamination from: air, anticoagulant, flush solution, or venous blood.
Sample obtained without clotting from: improper anticoagulant, improper mixing, or air exposure.

Sample analyzed within: 15 minutes (room temperature), 60 minutes (iced at 4°C).

---

1) ABG sampling is blood drawn, via puncture or A-line, from a peripheral artery to measure PaO$_2$, PaCO$_2$, pH, Hgb total, CoHgb, and/or MetHgb.
2) Adapted from AARC Clinical Practice Guideline: Sampling for Arterial Blood Gas Analysis, *Respiratory Care*, Volume 37, #8, 1992

ABG INTERPRETATION =

Classification

+

Calculations

+

Confirmation

A) Classification

Respiratory Acidosis	Respiratory Alkalosis	Metabolic Acidosis	Metabolic Alkalosis

B) Calculations

Calculate Compensation and Gaps:

Determines whether or not the body is compensating and whether or not other primary disorders exist.

Determine Oxygenation Status

C) Confirmation

Consistency with patient assessment, patient's baseline and check for accuracy: Determines validity of Classification and Calculations

---

KEYS to INTERPRETATION

1. Initial Technical Classification DOES NOT always equal a definitive ABG interpretation
2. Calculations are always ESSENTIAL
3. Patient assessment is ESSENTIAL
3. Patient BASELINE VALUES are often invaluable
4. Always check for POSSIBLE INACCURACIES in the gas result
5. SERIAL ABGs are often more important than a single ABG
6. ABG interpretation often leads to LIFE and DEATH decisions. Errors in interpretation can lead to dire consequences.

STEPS OF ABG INTERPRETATION

A) Classification   (See chart next page)

Primary Problem
Step 1. Check pH – Acidemia or Alkalemia?

Primary Cause
Step 2. Check PaCO₂ – is Respiratory the primary cause?

Step 3. Check HCO₃ – is Metabolic the primary cause?

Compensation
Step 4. Is the body compensating?

Initial Classification
Step 5. Technical Classification

B) Calculations

Step 6. Determine compensation and other primary causes

	PaCO₂	pH	HCO₃
Respiratory Acidosis			
Acute	↑ 10	↓ 0.08	↑ 1
Chronic	↑ 10	↓ 0.03	↑ 4
Respiratory Alkalosis			
Acute	↓ 10	↑ 0.08	↓ 2
Chronic	↓ 10	↑ 0.03	↓ 5

	HCO₃	pH	PaCO₂
Metabolic Acidosis	↓ 1	↓ 0.015	↓ 1.2
Metabolic Alkalosis	↑ 1	↑ 0.015	↑ 0.7

Step 7. Determine Anion Gap and Bicarbonate Gap

a. Anion Gap: $AG = Na - (Cl + HCO_3)$

b. Bicarbonate Gap (if an AG acidosis):

$$BG = Patient's\ HCO_3 + \Delta\ AG$$

BG Norm = 24 = AG Metabolic Acidosis

< 20 = AG Metabolic Acidosis + Non AG Metabolic Acidosis

> 28 = AG Metabolic Acidosis + Metabolic Alkalosis

Step 8. Determine Oxygenation (See page 2-2)

C) Confirmation

Step 9. Assess Patient

Step 10. Check for Accuracy (errors)

Step 11. **Final Interpretation**

CLASSIFICATION OF ABGs

Primary Problem	Primary Cause				Compensation	
Step 1: Check pH	**Step 2:** Check PaCO2 (N: 35-45)	Is Respiratory 1°?	**Step 3:** Check HCO3 (N: 22-26)	Is Metabolic 1°?	**Step 4:** Is the body compensating? (Yes/No)	**Step 5:** Technical Classification (1)
Alkalemia >7.45*	↑		↑	Yes	Yes (↑ PaCO2)	PC Metabolic Alkalosis
	N		↑	Yes	-	Metabolic Alkalosis (UC)
	↓	Yes	↑	Yes	-	Mixed Respiratory Alkalosis & Metabolic Alkalosis
	↓	Yes	N,↓		(3)	Respiratory Alkalosis (UC)
	↓	Yes	↓		Yes (↓ HCO3)	PC Respiratory Alkalosis
Normal 7.35-7.45	↑	Yes or compensat.?	↑	Yes or compensat?	Yes (↑ PaCO2)	FC Metabolic Alkalosis (7.41 - 7.45)
					Yes (↑ HCO3)	FC Respiratory Acidosis (7.35 - 7.39)
	N	N	N		-	Normal or Mixed Disorder (2)
	↓	Yes or compensating?	↓	Yes or compensating?	Yes (↓ PaCO2)	FC Metabolic Acidosis (7.35 - 7.39)
					Yes (↓ HCO3)	FC Respiratory Alkalosis (7.41 - 7.45)

		Acidemia < 7.35 **			
↑		Yes	↑	Yes (↑ HCO_3)	PC Respiratory Acidosis
↑	↑	Yes	N, ↑	(3)	Respiratory Acidosis (UC)
↑	↑	Yes	→	-	Mixed Respiratory & Metabolic Acidosis
N		Yes	→	-	Metabolic Acidosis (UC)
→		Yes	→	Yes (↓ $PaCO_2$)	PC Metabolic Acidosis

NOTES

(1) Technical classification terminology:

UC = Uncompensated (no compensation has occurred). Common usage leaves this designation off.

PC = Partially Compensated (pH has returned part way back to normal range)

FC = Fully Compensated (pH has returned back to normal range)

(2) Mixed Disorder (opposite disorders) = Respiratory acidosis & metabolic alkalosis or respiratory alkalosis & metabolic acidosis

($PaCO_2$ and HCO_3 go in same direction and "apparent compensation" is greater than expected)

(3) The immediate change in HCO_3 from normal is due to the hydrolysis effect, rather than compensation.

* As pH moves towards 7.8 = ↑ CNS stimulation: irritability, arrhythmias, tetany, convulsions, respiratory arrest, death. Definitive therapy is indicated at pH > 7.6.

** As pH moves towards 7.0 = ↓ CNS stimulation: drowsiness, lethargy, coma, death. Definitive therapy is often considered at pH < 7.15.

2-6

ABG Disorders

Technical Class.	Functional Class.	Compensation Status
UC Respiratory Acidosis	Acute Respiratory Acidosis	**Kidneys:** Either not enough time to begin compensation or the kidneys are compromised
PC Respiratory Acidosis	Chronic Respiratory Acidosis	**Kidneys:** Either not enough time to fully compensate or compensation is maximal (chronic), but pH not back to normal range
FC Respiratory Acidosis	Chronic Respiratory Acidosis	**Kidneys:** Compensation is maximal (chronic) and full – pH is back to normal range (occurs only in very mild disorders)
UC Respiratory Alkalosis	Acute Respiratory Alkalosis	**Kidneys:** Either not enough time to begin compensation or kidneys are compromised
PC Respiratory Alkalosis	Chronic Respiratory Alkalosis	**Kidneys:** Either not enough time to fully compensate or compensation is maximal (chronic), but pH not back to normal range
FC Respiratory Alkalosis	Chronic Respiratory Alkalosis	**Kidneys:** Compensation is maximal (chronic) and full –pH is back to normal range (occurs in most disorders)
UC Metabolic Acidosis	Metabolic Acidosis*	**Respiratory** system is compromised (rare that there is zero compensation) or such a mild change in HCO_3 that any change in $PaCO_2$ is minimal.
PC Metabolic Acidosis	Metabolic Acidosis	**Respiratory:** Compensation is usually immediate and maximal, but is not back to normal range
FC Metabolic Acidosis	Metabolic Acidosis	**Respiratory:** This classification essentially *does not exist* because $PaCO_2$ generally does not return pH back to normal range. If pH is normal, there is usually a secondary respiratory disorder at work.
UC Metabolic Alkalosis	Metabolic Alkalosis	**Respiratory** : If there is no compensation, there is usually a secondary respiratory alkalosis
PC Metabolic Alkalosis	Metabolic Alkalosis	**Respiratory:** Compensation is usually immediate and maximal, but pH is not back to normal range
FC Metabolic Alkalosis	Metabolic Alkalosis	**Respiratory:** This class. really *does not exist* because $PaCO_2$ generally does not return pH back to normal range. If pH is normal, there is usually a secondary respiratory disorder at work.

NOTES

Technical classification terminology:

UC = Uncompensated (no compensation has occurred). Common usage leaves this designation off.

PC = Partially Compensated (pH has returned part way back to normal range)

FC = Fully Compensated (pH has returned back to normal range)

A *corrected* blood gas disorder is one in which the pH is returned to normal range by altering the component primarily affected.

A *compensated* blood gas disorder is one in which the pH is returned towards normal range by altering the component not primarily affected.

Because of the limitations of the lungs or kidneys to "fully" compensate for most alterations of each other (i.e., completely return pH to normal), "full" or "complete" compensation is more appropriately referred to as "maximal" compensation.

Maximal Compensation = the body has completely compensated all it is designed to compensate – usually pH returns only 50% of the way back.

If the disorder is *mild*, maximal compensation may return the pH to within normal range, resulting in a "full" compensation (FC).

If the disorder is *moderate to severe*, maximal compensation will only return the pH part way back to normal range, resulting in a "partial" compensation (PC).

* The terms "acute" and "chronic" for metabolic disorders are often omitted because, *functionally*, there is usually no time distinction between acute and chronic metabolic disorders – the respiratory system compensation is usually immediate. Also, because all metabolic disorders are essentially Partially Compensated, all metabolic disorders are simply termed Metabolic Acidosis or Metabolic Alkalosis, without any further descriptive terminology.

Functional Classification = common usage and function.

2-8

See Oakes' ABG Pocket Guide: Interpretation and Management for details on each ABG Disorder, Including:
- Respiratory Acidosis, Respiratory Alkalosis, Metabolic Acidosis, Metabolic Alkalsosis
- Quick Reference Charts for determining Compensation
- Signs and Symptoms
- Physiological Effects and Clinical Manifestations
- Causes and Management
- Calculating Anion Gaps
- Calculating Bicarbonate Gaps
- Diagnosing Double and Triple Disorders
- Interpreting ABG's in COPD Patients
- Hypoxic Drive Theory

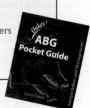

See Equation Chapter for a Complete List of Acid-Base Equations

See Respiratory Procedures, Chapter 10 for extensive Oxygenation information, including assessment, interpretation, devices, and more.

1. Check Patient – Does ABG line up with patient's clinical condition?
  Good gases & patient in distress; Bad gases & no patient distress?
  Rising or normal $PaCO_2$ in severe respiratory distress (e.g., asthma)?

2. Check Lab Values

  HCO_3 should be within 1-2 mEq/L of Total CO_2
  A difference of > 4 mEq/L = technical error

  Actual HCO_3 should = 24 x $PaCO_2$/ (80 - last two digits of pH)
  (only works for pH between 7.30 – 7.50)

3. Check for Errors
  A) Sampling Errors
    1) Venous blood or contamination with venous blood ($\downarrow PaO_2$,
      $\uparrow PaCO_2$, $\downarrow$ pH).
      Venous $PaO_2 \approx 40$ (or does not match patient clinical
      condition; cross check with SpO_2)
    2) Air in sample – Effect varies with agitation, duration, temp, &
      volume.
      (PaO_2 higher than expected; $PaCO_2$ lower than expected)

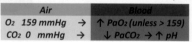

Air		Blood
O_2 159 mmHg	$\rightarrow$	$\uparrow PaO_2$ (unless > 159)
CO_2 0 mmHg	$\rightarrow$	$\downarrow PaCO_2 \rightarrow \uparrow$ pH

    This can result in a negative PA-aO2!
    3) Anticoagulant (heparin) - too much (rare today, but same
      effect as air.)
    4) Patient not on reported FIO_2
    5) Patient not in a steady state (ABG too soon after a change in
      FIO_2 or MV)

  B) Measuring Errors
    1) Improper calibration, quality control, or sample mixing
    2) Documentation/transcription errors ($PaCO_2$/PaO_2 reversed?
      orally conveyed?)
    3) Wrong patient blood
    4) Time delay in measuring (> 30 min. un-iced; > 60 min. iced)
    5) $\uparrow$ WBC or platelets $\rightarrow$ $\downarrow PaO_2$ (leukocyte larceny)

4. Check PaO2 – FIO2 Relationship
  A) On room air: PaO_2 should be < 130 mmHg
  B) On $\uparrow FIO_2$: PaO_2 should be < 5 x FIO_2
        (Example: FIO_2 0.4; PaO_2 should be < 200)
  C) Always question: Was mask on patient, cannula in nose, etc.?

5. Check PaO2/SaO2 – SpO2 relationship (See page 10-76)

3   CHEST X-RAY INTERPRETATION

Keys to Good CXR Interpretation

1. **Be Systematic.**
   Regardless of the system you adopt, review every CXR in the same order, every time. Otherwise, you may miss something critical.

2. **Be Aware.**
   The CXR must be interpreted in context of the patient's status. Avoid treating an X-Ray, "just because it looks bad," but use it as another tool.

3. **Be Weary.**
   Use caution in making decisions (such as pulling back an Endotracheal Tube) based solely upon a CXR. Body habitus, poor quality, and other factors can make locating tubes difficult at times.

CXR

PARAMETERS TO CHECK

A	Airways	Trachea (midline?, ET-tube), carina, periphery (air bronchograms)
B	Bones	Fractures, kyphoscoliosis, rib spacing
C	Cardiac	Heart width (<1/2 thorax), silhouette sign
D	Diaphragm	R higher than L, elevated, flat
E	Esophagus	
F	Fissures	Minor, major
G	Gastric	Gastric bubble
H	Hila	L higher than R, enlargement
I	Interstitial	Alveolar vs. interstitial, ↑ by breast
J	Junction lines	
K	Kerley B lines	Right base = CHF, A&C lines
L	Lobes	Collapse, hyperaerated, infiltrates
M	Mediastinum	Air
N	Nodules	Air-filled, location, size
O	Over-aeration	Asthma, blebs, emphysema, foreign objects, MV, tension pneumothorax
P	Pleura	Air, costophrenic blunting
Q	Quickly	Examine name plate, name, date, time
R	Respiration	I = diaphragm ↓ to 6 anterior, 10 posterior E = ↑ heart size, ↓ volume, ↑interstitium
S	Segments	See Pg 3-6
T	Tubes/lines	ET tube, catheters (CVP, Swans, etc.)
U	Under-perfusion	Westermark (↓ pulmonary marking due to emboli or PA catheter)
V	Volume	R = 55%, L = 45%
W	Women	Breast shadows (also in obese males)
X	Xtra densities	Foreign bodies

CXR

Reprinted with permission and adapted from Sheldon, R.L.: Chapter 19. In Scanlon, C.L. et. al., editors: *Egan's Fundamentals of Respiratory Therapy*, 6th Ed. copyright 1995 by Mosby Yearbook, Inc., St Louis.

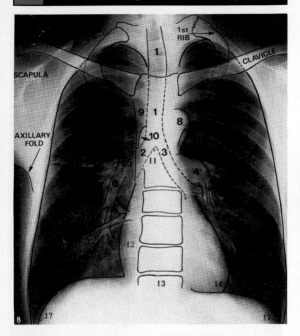

NORMAL CXR (PA PROJECTION)

1. trachea
2. right mainstem
3. left mainstem
4. left pulmonary artery
5. right upper lobe pulmonary vein
6. right interlobar artery
7. right upper and lower lobe vein
8. aortic knob
9. superior vena cava
10. ascending aorta
11. carina
12. right atrium
13. right ventricle
14. left ventricle
15. left hemidiaphragm
16. right hemidiaphragm
17. costophrenic angle
18. minor fissure

Reprinted with permission from Fraser, R.H. and Pare, J.A.: *Organ Physiology: Structure and Function of the Lung*. Copyright 1977 by W.B Saunders, Co., Philadelphia

3-3

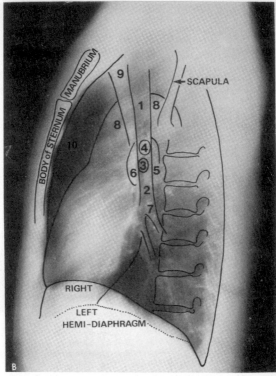

1. trachea
2. right intermediate bronchus
3. left upper lobe bronchus
4. right upper lobe bronchus
5. left interlobar artery
6. right interlobar artery
7. pulmonary veins
8. aortic arch
9. brachiocephalic vessels
10. substernal space

Reprinted with permission from Fraser, R.H. and Pare, J.A.: *Organ Physiology: Structure and Function of the Lung.* Copyright 1977 by W.B Saunders, Co., Philadelphia

ABNORMAL APPEARANCES/CAUSES

Appearances	Possible Causes
Air Bronchogram – Can visualize airways out towards the periphery	Usually occurs with consolidated alveoli
AP vs. PA Projection – AP usually shows ↓ lung volumes, elevated hemi-diaphragms, ↑ lung marking in bases, heart enlarged, scapula overlies upper fields, often rotated	Portable x-ray, AP usually taken for bed-ridden patients (esp. while on MV)
Butterfly Pattern: Puffy cloudiness in central lung fields	Pulmonary edema
Honeycomb cloudiness throughout lung fields	Interstitial edema
Costophrenic Blunting – Rounded angle	Fluid in pleural space
↑ Heart Size: RV – Pulmonary artery pushed towards L cardiac border	Cor pulmonale
RA	Cor pulmonale
LV – Rounding of L cardiac border and boot-shaped extension	CHF
LA – Lateral projection of R cardiac border	CHF
Kerley B Lines – Perpendicular lines to pleura in peripheral bases	Interstitial edema
Miliary Pattern – Small, round regular densities	Alveolar filling with fluid or material
Nodular Pattern – Confluent densities of different sizes	↑ Interstitial or alveolar pattern
↓ Peripheral Markings – ↓ or absent markings in periphery	Air in pleural space, pulmonary hypertension, pulmonary embolism
Dilated Pulmonary Arteries – Antler-shaped, cloudiness at base	Pulmonary hypertension
Reticular Pattern – Irregular network of straight or curved densities	Interstitial infiltrates or fibrosis
Reticulogranular Pattern – Ground glass appearance	ARDS

Silhouette Sign – Loss of the normal silhouette of the heart, aorta, or diaphragm (*See below*)	Water density (infiltrates) in anatomic contact with heart, aorta, or diaphragm
Volume ↓ – ↓ Size of thoracic cage, elevated diaphragms, ↑ interstitial markings	Atelectasis, ↓ surfactant, ↓ CL
Volume ↑ – ↑ size of thoracic cage (hyper-aeration), flattened diaphragm, ↓ interstitial markings	*Trapped air:* asthma, emphysema, ↑MV volumes, ↑ PEEP or auto-PEEP, tension pneumothorax

*See Chapter 11 for X-ray appearance of specific diseases and disorders

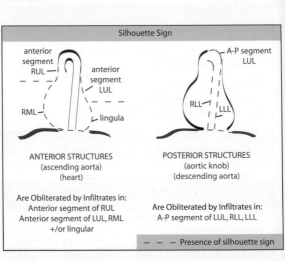

Silhouette Sign

ANTERIOR STRUCTURES
(ascending aorta)
(heart)

Are Obliterated by Infiltrates in:
Anterior segment of RUL
Anterior segment of LUL, RML
+/or lingular

POSTERIOR STRUCTURES
(aortic knob)
(descending aorta)

Are Obliterated by Infiltrates in:
A-P segment of LUL, RLL, LLL

– – – Presence of silhouette sign

This diagram shows the relative location of infiltrates as they appear on a Chest X-Ray (CXR). Knowing this may aid in positioning for postural drainage.

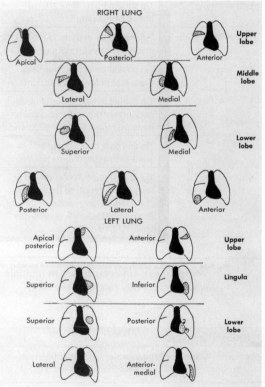

Reprinted with permission from Sheldon, R.L..In Scanlan, C.L., Spearman, C.B. and Sheldon, R.L., editors: *Egan's Fundamentals of Respiratory Therapy*, 6th ed. Copyright 1995 by the Mosby Yearbook, Inc., St. Louis

Common Chest X-Ray Findings by Disease/Disorder -
See individual disease/disorder in Disease Chapter

Approximate Tube/Line Placement on CXR

Line/Tube	Placement
Endotracheal Tube	Tip should be midline 2-6 cm above carina (adult)
Tracheostomy Tube	Tip should be midline 1/2 to 1/3 distance between stoma/carina
CVP Line	Tip should be in Superior Vena Cava, just before Right Atrium
PA Catheter	Tip should in right or left Pulmonary Artery (about 5 cm distal to main pulmonary artery bifurcation)
NG or OG Tube	Tip and side hole should be beyond gastroesophageal junction
Chest Tube	Tip of Radiopaque line should be within the pleural space and medial to the inner margin of the ribs Positioning depends on whether collecting air or fluid

Verify Tube or Line placement in multiple ways - do not rely solely on the CXR.

Additional Resources

See Oakes' **RespiratoryUpdate.com** for further information and explanations of CXR Interpretation, including direct links to:

4 ECG INTERPRETATION

How To Read An ECG

1. Check for calibration (10mm high box with strip moving 25 mm/sec) and assess for artifact.
2. Measure ventricular rate (See below)
3. Check P wave (Shape, position, and # = atrial rate)
4. Measure P-R interval (Normal = 0.12 - 0.20 seconds)
5. Evaluate QRS shape and interval (Normal < 0.12 seconds)
6. Check regularity of waves (the distance between R-R waves should not vary > 0.12 seconds)
7. Evaluate T wave and ST segment (See Pg 4-10)

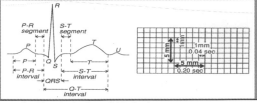

Measuring Ventricular Rate: 2 Methods

1. **Irregular rhythms (or slow)**: Count # R waves (in 6 seconds, i.e., two 3 sec intervals or 2 boxes) X 10 = rate/min
2. **Regular Rhythms**: "Rule of 300": Count # of large boxes between R waves (start with 1 on a red line). Divide 300 by the # of boxes.

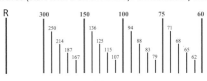

ECG

4-1

Standard ECG Leads

	Limb		Chest
Positive Electrode			
I	Left arm	V1	R of sternum in 4th ICS
II	Left leg	V2	L of sternum in 4th ICS
III	Left leg	V3	Midway between V2 and V4
aVR	Right arm	V4	Midclavicular line in 5th ICS
aVL	Left arm	V5	Anterior axillary, same level as V4
aVF	Left leg	V6	Midaxillary line, same level as V4

Negative Electrode	
I	Right arm
II	Right arm
III	Left arm

TROUBLESHOOTING

Problem in:	Check Leads:
VI-V6	Chest lead that corresponds to tracing
Lead I	LA, RA
Lead II	LL, RA
Lead III	LL, LA
aVR	RA, LA, LL
aVL	LA, RA, LL
aVF	LL, RA, LA

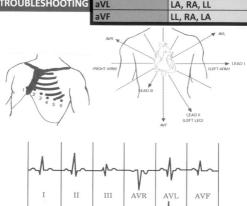

ECG

Interpreting ECGs: According to Rate

Normal	Slow	Fast
Sinus rhythm	Sinus bradycardia	Sinus tachycardia
Sinus arrhythmia	(< 60/min)	(>100/min)
SA block	AV nodal rhythm	PAT (150-250)
Wandering	(40-60/min)	Atrial flutter
pacemaker	2nd ° AV block	(250-350)
PAC	(1/2 to 1/3 atrial rate)	Atrial fib (350-450)
PNC	3rd ° AV block	AV nodal tach
1st ° AV block	(< 40/min)	(150-250)
PVC	V-fib (0/min)	V-tach (150-250)
	V standstill (0/min)	

According to P Wave

	Absent	Buried	Abnormal	Inverted
Wandering pacemaker		X	X	
PAC			X	X
PAT		X	X	
Atrial Flutter			X	
A-fib	X		X	
PNC		X		X
AV nodal tachycardia		X		X
AV nodal rhythm		X		X
PVC	X			
V-tach	X			

According to Prolonged PR Intervals

P with every QRS	1st ° Heart Block
Progressive PR prolongation	2nd ° Heart Block (Type I)
Constant PR with dropped beats	2nd ° Heart Block (Type II)
No relation between P and QRS	3rd ° Heart Block

Classification of Cardiac Arrhythmias (by Prognosis)

Minor Arrhythmias		Major Arrhythmias
Sinus Tachycardia	PAC (> 6/min)	Sinoatrial Arrest
Sinus Bradycardia	Atrial Tachycardia	1st ° Heart Block
Sinus Arrhythmia	Atrial Flutter	2nd ° Heart Block
PAC (< 6/min)	Atrial Fibrillation	3rd ° Heart Block
PVC (< 6/min)	PVC (> 6/min)	Bundle Branch Block
PNC (< 6/min)	AV Nodal Rhythm	
Wandering Pacemaker		

Death Producing: Ventricular Tachycardia / Fibrillation / Standstill

Summary of Basic Arrhythmias (according to site of origin)

Type	Identifying Features	Appearance (Lead II)	Clinical Notes
SA Node			
Normal Sinus Rhythm	Rate: 60-100/min, P waves regular P-R regular (0.12-0.20), QRS regular (< 0.12), R-R regular, T wave upright and round, ST segment is flat		Normal Rhythm
Sinus Arrhythmia	↓ R-R interval on inspiration, irregular rhythm		Probably vagal stimulation from pressures in thorax, benign, no Tx needed
Sinus Tachycardia	Rate > 100/min		Causes – Fever, hypoxemia, ↓BP, hypovolemia, pain, sepsis, heart failure, bronchodilators. May lead to ischemia.
Sinus Bradycardia	Rate < 60/min		Causes – Carotid massage, hypothermia, Valsalva, tracheal Sx. May lead to ↓BP/CO, syncope, CHF, shock.
Sinus (SA) Block (arrest)	Entire beat absent		Also called Sino-atrial arrest or escape.
Wandering Pacemaker	Rate varies, P waves vary in shape & position, P-R interval varies		Rate >100 = Multifocal Atrial Tachycardia (MAT). Seen in COPD or digitalis toxicity.

4-4

Type	Identifying Features	Appearance (Lead II)	
Atrial			
Premature Atrial Contractions (PAC)	Premature P waves (abnormal or inverted), short T-P interval before beat, long T-P after beat		May confuse with Premature Nodal Contraction.
Premature Atrial Tachycardia (PAT, PSVT)	Rate 150-250/min, P waves abnormal or buried. Called supraventricular tach (SVT) and may be parcxsymal.		Sudden onset and termination. Patients may experience lightheadedness or palpitations. May lead to ↓BP/CO, myocardial ischemia, CHF.
Atrial Flutter	Atrial rate 250-350/min, ventricular rate normal, sawtooth P waves, 2:1, 3:1, 4:1 block of QRS		Commonly associated with pulmonary disease. May return to normal or deteriorate to A-fib. ↑ risk for embolism.
Atrial Fibrillation (A-fib)	No clear P waves, atrial rate 350-430/min, irregulatr ventricular rhythm		Often asymptomatic, except ↓ cardiac reserve. ↑ risk for embolism.
Nodal			
Premature Nodal Contractions	P wave absent or inverted after the QRS		PJC (or PNC) = Premature junctional complex May confuse with PAC

Type	Identifying Features	Appearance (Lead II)	Clinical Notes
Paroxysmal Junctional (A-V nodal) Tachycardia	Rate 150-250/min, P wave variable		
A-V Nodal (Junctional) Rhythm	Rate 40-60/min, P waves absent or inverted		Also called junctional escape or idio-junctional rhythm.
1st ° A-V Heart Block	Constant, prolonged P-R interval (> 0.2 sec)		Often asymptomatic. May be misread as a normal sinus rhythm
2nd ° A-V Heart Block (Type I, Wenckebach)	Progressively longer P-R interval until a beat is dropped		Often asymptomatic
2nd ° A-V Heart Block (Type II)	Some non-conducted P waves (no QRS), constant P-R intervals, slow ventricular rate		May lead to ↓ BP/CO, weakness, and fainting. Also called Mobitz II
3rd ° A-V Heart Block (Complete)	No relationship between P waves and QRS, atrial rate normal		Atria and ventricles beat independently (A-V dissociation). Rate 40 – 60/min = Junctional rhythm Rate < 40/min = Ventricular rhythm

4-6

Type	Identifying Features	Appearance (Lead II)	Clinical Notes
Bundle Branch Block (R or L)	QRS widened (>/= 0.12) with rabbit-ear feature		Appearance highly variable Cause: underlying heart disease
Ventricular			
Premature Ventricular Contractions (PVC)	Premature, wide (> 0.12), distorted QRS with no P wave, T wave opposite, full compensatory pause		> 6/min is pathological. Most common cause is myocardial ischemia. May be caused by anxiety, ↓K+, excessive caffeine, or medications. R-on-T may lead to V-tach.
Bigeminy = 1 normal coupled with 1 PVC Trigeminy = 2 normal coupled with 1 PVC Unifocal = 2 or more PVCs that look alike (same heart site) Multifocal = 2 or more PVCs that look different (different sites)		Couplet = 2 PVCs side by side Triplet = 3 PVCs in a row	
Ventricular Tachycardia (V-Tach*)	Series of PVCs (>3 in row), rate 150-250/min		May quickly lead to ↓BP/CO, V-fib, loss of consciousness, and death.
Ventricular Flutter	Series of smooth sine waves, rate 250-350/min		May quickly lead to ↓BP/CO, V-fib, loss of consciousness, and death

4-7

Type	Identifying Features	Appearance (Lead II)	Clinical Notes
Torsades de Pointes	a form of VTach where QRS complex varies beat-to-beat, ventricular rate 150-250. May change from + to - axis.		May return to NSR or become more serious. Treat with ACLS algorithm for VTach.
Ventricular Fibrillation (V-fib) *	No well defined, erratic QRS, rate 350-450/min		Rhythm may be mistaken for either V-tach or asystole. Immediate ↓CO →coma. Treat with defibrillation.
Ventricular Standstill (Asystole) *	Essentially a flat line		Caution: a simple disconnect of ECG lead can resemble asystole. Check for immediate pulselessness, ↓ BP, and loss of consciousness.
Pulseless Electrical Activity (PEA)	Any heart rhythm that should be producing a palpable pulse, but is not.	Appearance Varies, Treat underlying cause: H (hypovolemia, hypoxia, hypo/hyperkalemia, hypothermia) D (drug overdose) T (tamponade, tension pneumothorax, thromboses) Most Common: resp. failure due to hypoxia	

ECG's must be interpreted in light of the patient's clinical symptoms, physical exam, medications, electrolyte balance, body size, and age. Interpretation should not be made solely on the basis of the ECG findings.

4-8

Interpreting Abnormalities *

Pulmonary Effects

COPD	Pulmonary Embolism (→ Cor Pulmonale)
Low voltage in all leads, Rt. axis deviation, MAT	S1Q3⊥3 = Wide S in I, large Q in III, inverted T in III and V1-V4. ST depressed in II, often transient RBBB

Cardiac Hypertrophy

Atrial Hypertrophy: P waves more than 3 small squares wide	
Right Atrial	**Left Atrial**
In VI - Large, diphasic P wave with tall initial component	In VI - Large diphasic P wave with wide terminal component

Ventricular Hypertrophy	
Right Ventricular	**Left Ventricular**
R wave > S wave(VI) R wave progressively smaller (VI→ V6). S wave persists in V5 and V6. Wide QRS and right axis deviation	S wave (VI) + R wave (V5) = > 35 mm L axis deviat., wide QRS T wave slants down slowly and returns up rapidly (inverted) (V5 or 6)

Electrolytes

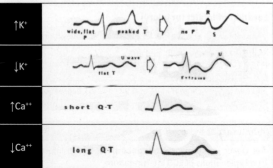

↑K⁺	wide, flat P	peaked T	◇	no P	R S
↓K⁺	flat T	U wave	◇	Extreme	U
↑Ca⁺⁺	short Q-T				
↓Ca⁺⁺	long Q-T				

Cardiac Ischemia, Injury or Infarction

Acute

Ischemia = Inverted T Wave

Inverted T wave is symmetrical (V2-V6).
Signifies an acute process and usually lasts only a few hours.

Injury = Elevated ST segment

Signifies an acute process and usually lasts only a few hours. If T wave is also elevated off baseline, suspect pericarditis. Location of injury may be determined like infarct location.
ST depression = digitalis, subendocardial infarct or exercise stress test.

Acute or Chronic

Infarction = Q Wave

Insignificant (small) Q waves may be normal (esp. V5 and V6).
Significant (abnormal) Q waves must be > one small square (0.04sec) wide or > 1/3 QRS height in lead III.

Location of Infarct (or injury)

Anterior	Q wave in V1,V2,V3 or V4 (ST elevation)
Inferior	Q in II, III, and aVF
Lateral	Q in I and aVL
Posterior	Large R in V1 and V2 (ST depression) Mirror test

Additional Resources

See Oakes' **RespiratoryUpdate.com** for further information and explanations of ECG Interpretation.

5   LABORATORY TESTS

!

    Selected tests related to Respiratory Care follow, with commonly used values. Normal values are variable between institutions and the method used, and values of healthy vs. diseased patients may overlap. Drugs and iatrogenic factors are not listed as causes of abnormal values, but should always be considered.

Danger Levels

Electrolytes	Low	
Na+	< 120 mEq/L	> 160 mEq/L
K+	< 2.5 mEq/L	> 6.5 mEq/L
Hematology		
Hematocrit	< 14%	> 60%
WBC	< 2000 uL	> 50,000 uL
Platelets	< 20,000 uL	> 1,00,000 uL
PT	> 40 sec	
Blood & Serum		
pH	< 7.20	> 7.60
PaCO2	< 20 mmHg	> 60 mmHg
PaO2	< 40 mmHg	> 100 mmHg (newborn)
HCO3	< 10 mEq/L	> 40 mEq/L
Glucose	< 40 mg/dL	> 400 mg/dL

Electrolytes

Test	Normal Value	Clinical Significance	Clinical Increases	Clinical Decreases
Na⁺ (Sodium)	135-145 mEq/L SI 135-145 mmol/L	Major extracellular cation, comprises majority of osmotically active solute. Greatly affects distribution of body water.	↑ *Na+* – Cushings syndrome, hyperadrenocorticism, excessive intake. ↓ *Body H₂O* – Dehydration, hyperpnea, diabetes, diuretics, cardiac failure. *S & S* – Thirst, viscous mucous, dry, rough tongue.	↓ *Na* (with ↓ body H₂O) – adrenal insufficiency, alkali, burns, diuretics, dehydration, trauma. ↑ *Body H₂O* – ↓ renal output, artificial hyperglycemia, CHF, cirrhosis, inappropriate ADH, renal insufficiency. *S & S* – ↑ HR, ↑ BP, cold, clammy skin, apprehension, convulsions.
K⁺	3.5-5.0 mEq/L SI 3.5-5.0 mmol/L	Major intracellular cation, maintains intracellular osmolality, affects muscle contraction, plays role in nerve impulses, enzyme action, cell membrane function.	*Excessive administration* *Shift from cells* – Acidosis (metabolic), infection, succinylcholine, trauma. ↓ *renal output* *S&S* – Arrhythmias, muscle weakness.	*Shift into cells* – Alkalosis *GI loss* – anorexia, diarrhea, NG Sx, vomiting. ↑ *renal output* – Cushings syndrome, diabetic ketoacidosis, diuretics, renal tubular-acidosis, steroid therapy. *S&S* – Arrhythmias, muscle weak
Cl⁻ (Chloride)	95-105 mEq/L SI 95-105 mmol/L	Principle extracellular anion, important in acid-base balance	Cardiac decompensation, renal insufficiency, salt intake	COPD, Cushings syndrome, dehydration, diabetic ketoacidosis, diuretics, fever, metab acidosis, pneumonia

Test	Normal Value	Clinical Significance	Clinical Increases	Clinical Decreases
$PO_4^{=}$	1.4-2.7 mEq/L SI 0.9-1.5 mmcl/L	Major intracellular anion	Renal insufficiency	Diabetic ketoacidosis
Ca++ (Calcium)	4.5-5.8 mEq/L SI 2.1-2.6mmol/L	Essential anion for bones, teeth, mucoproteins Role in cell membrane, muscle contraction and coagulation	Acidosis, adrenal insufficiency, diuretics (thiazide), immobilization, sarcoidosis, tumors.	Alkalosis, diarrhea, hypoproteinemia, osteomalacia, renal insufficiency, steroid therapy, vitamin D deficiency.
Mg++	1.3-2.5 mEq/L SI 0.8-1.3 mmol/L	Intracellular cation, important in ATP function, acetylcholine release at N-M junction.	Antacid ingestion, parathyroidectomy, renal insufficiency	Chronic alcoholism, diabetic acidosis, diarrhea, NG Sx, severe renal disease

Hematology

Test	Normal Value	Clinical Significance	Clinical Increases	Clinical Decreases
Erythrocytes (RBCs)	Male 4.6-6.2 million/μL SI 4.6-6.2 10^{12}/L Female 4.2-5.4 million/μL SI 4.2-5.4 10^{12}/L	Number of cells available to carry O_2/CO_2	1° polycythemia 2° polycythemia from chronic hypoxemia, severe diarrhea and dehydration	Anemias, leukemia, hemorrhage followed by restored blood volume
Hemoglobin (Hgb)	Male 13-18 gm/dL SI 8.1-11.2 mmol/L Female 12-16 gm/dL SI 7.4-9.9 mmol/L	Grams of hemoglobin in 100 mL of whole blood	Polycythemia, CHF, COPD, dehydration, high altitudes.	Acute blood loss, anemias, ↑ fluid intake, pregnancy

5-3

Test	Normal Value	Clinical Significance	Clinical Increases	Clinical Decreases
Hematocrit (Hct)	Male 39-55% SI 0.39-0.55 Female 36-48% SI 0.36-0.48	% blood volume occupied by RBCs	COPD, dehydration, erythrocytosis, shock.	Acute blood loss, anemias, ↑ fluid intake, pregnancy
Reticulocytes	Male 0.5-2.7% of RBCs Female 0.5-4.1% of RBCs SI 0.005-0.015	A young RBC	↑ bone marrow activity, blood loss, infection, polycythemia (Ruba vera)	↓ bone marrow activity, leukemia, severe anemia, aplastic anemia
RBC Sedimentation Rate	Male 0-15 mm/hr Female 0-20 mm/hr SI same	↑rate = progression of inflammation and destructive disease	Active syphillis, acute infection, menstruation, MI, pregnancy, shock, TB, tissue destruction	Allergies, CHF, fibrinogen deficiency (will be 0), newborns, polycythemia, sickle cell
RDW	11.5% - 14.5%	Size (width) differences of RBCs.	Early indicator of anemia: iron-deficiency; folic acid deficiency; pernicious or sickle cell anemia	N/A

Test	Normal Value	Clinical Significance		Clinical Decreases
Leukocytes (WBCs)	Total: 5,000 - 10,000 / uL SI 5-10 x 10^9/L	Blood cells which fight infection	Leukocytosis: acute infections, post surgery, trauma.	Leukopenia: L shift (more immature), cancer therapy, overwhelmed or suppressed immune system.
Neutrophils (segs/bands)	40-75%		Bacterial infection, neoplasm, epinephrine, steroids	CHF, HIV, renal failure,
Lymphocytes	20-45%	T & B Cells	Chronic infection, viral infection (hepatitis, mono),TB.	
Monocytes	2-10%			
Eosinophils	1-6%		Allergy/collagen (asthma)	Steroid therapy
Basophils	0-1%			
Platelet Count	150,000-400,C00/μL SI 150-400 x 10^9/L	Blood constituent for clotting	COPD, high altitude, inflammation, malignancy, PE, TB, trauma, many drugs	Acute leukemia, anemias, bleeding, lupus, (many).
Bleeding Time	1-7 min (Ivy) SI 60-420 sec	Measure of platelet function	Aspirin, DIC, thrombocytopenia, uremia	
Thrombin Time	16-22 sec	Identifies prothrombin deficiency when BOTH PT and PTT are prolonged	Heparin contamination	
Prothrombin Time (PT)	10-14 sec	Extrinsic path: coumadin therapy	Clotting factor defect, liver disease, lupus erythymatosus	

5-5

Test	Normal Value	Clinical Significance	Clinical Increases	Clinical Decreases
Activated Partial Prothrombin Time (APPT)	25-39 sec Critical value >70 sec	Intrinsic path: heparin therapy monitor	Clotting factor defects, liver disease	

Chemistry

Test	Normal Value	Clinical Significance	Clinical Increases	Clinical Decreases
Acetoacetate (Acetone)	Negative	Indicator of Type 1 IDDM	Diabetic ketoacidosis	
Alpha 1- antitrypsin	< 200 mg/dL		Abcesses, arthritis, early inflammation, pneumonia.	COPD
Anion Gap	7-16 mEq/L	$Na+ - (Cl- + HCO_3)$	Keto or lactic acidosis, salicylate or ethylene glycol poison, dehydration.	Various dilutional states
Aspartate Amino Transferase (AST,SGOT)	10-40 U/mL SI 0.08-0.32 μmol/sec/L	Enzyme present in heart, liver and muscle - released with injury.	MI, liver disease, pulmonary infarct, skeletal muscle disease (see CPK)	Pregnancy
Bicarbonate (HCO³)	22-30 mEq/L SI 22-30 mmol/L	Major buffer of blood	Chronic respiratory acidosis, metabolic alkalosis(See ABGs)	Chronic respiratory alkalosis, metab. acidosis

Test	Normal Value	Clinical Significance	Clinical Increases	Clinical Decreases
BNP (b-type natriuretic peptide)	**Heart Failure:** 100-300 - Possible > 300 pg/mL - mild > 600 pg/mL - moderate > 900 pg/mL - severe	BNP is secreted from heart ventricles in response to Δ in Ht. when Ht. failure develops and worsens	Indicates heart failure	Decrease in patients taking drug therapy for heart failure, such as ACE inhibitors, beta blockers, and diuretics.
Creatine Kinase (CPK)	Male 38-174 U/L Female 26-140 U/L	Enzyme in heart, skeletal muscle	MI, muscle disease, severe exercise, polymyositis	Relative cardiac enzyme levels in blood following a myocardial infarction.
Creatine phospho-kinase MB Band (CPK-MB, CK-MB)	0% - 6%	Specific CK isoenzyme for heart muscle	Acute MI, severe angina pectoris, cardiac surgery, cardiac ischemia, myocarditis, hypokalemia, cardiac defibrillation	
Creatinine	0.6-1.5 mg/dL SI 53-133 μmol/L	By-product of muscle metabolism	Nephritis, renal insufficiency, urinary tract obstruction (Indicator of kidney function)	Debilitation
D-Dimer	0-500 ng/mL	fibrin fragments, adjunct test to rule out PE in some pts	PE, DVT, DIC, recent surgery, trauma, infection, liver disease, pregnancy, eclampsia, heart disease, and some CA	anticoagulant therapy (false negative)

5-7

Test	Normal Value	Clinical Significance	Clinical Increases	Clinical Decreases
Glucose	60-110 mg/dL (true) SI 3.5-5.5 mmol/L	Blood sugar	Diabetes mellitus, infections, stress, steroids, trauma, uremia	Adrenal insufficiency, insulin
HgbA$_{1c}$	Nondiabetic: 2-5% Diabetic control: 2.5-6% High average: 6.1-7.5% Diabetic uncontrol: > 8%	Long term (1-4 months) monitoring of glucose level in known diabetics	Diabetes (poorly controlled or uncontrolled), hyperglycemia, recently diagnosed diabetes mellitus, alcohol ingestion, hemodialysis	Pregnancy, chronic blood loss, chronic renal failure, hemolytic anemia, conditions that decreases red blood cell life span
Insulin	4-24 μU/mL SI 42-167 pmol/L	Pancreatic enzyme Regulates glucose metabolism	Acromegaly, insulinoma, obesity	Diabetes mellitus
Lactic Acid	5-20 mg/dL SI 0.5-1.6 mmol/L	By-product of an-aerobic metabolism	Hypoxia, CHF, ↑muscle activity, hemorrhage, shock	
Lactic Dehydrogenase (LDH)	Highly method dependent	Enzyme which catalyzes inter-conversion of lactic and pyruvate	5 Isoenzymes : Damaged cells: MI, muscle disease, liver disease, neoplastic disease, pulmonary infarction.	LDH1 > 2 = MI ↑LDH 1-5 = heart failure ↑LDH 2,3 = pulm. infarct ↑LDH 4,5 = kidney, liver ↑LDH 5 = liver disease

5-8

Test	Normal Value	Clinical Significance		Clinical Decreases
Protein	Total: 6-8 g/dL SI 60-80 gm/L Albumin: 3.5-5.5 gm/dL SI 35-55 gm/L Globulin: 1.5-3 gm/dL SI 15-30 gm/L	Blood proteins affecting colloidal pressure Defense proteins	Dehydration, shock Relative only Infections, erythmatosus, liver disease, lupus	Hemorrhage, liver disease, leukemia, malnutr, nephrosis, neoplastic disease. Agammaglobulimemia, leukemia,malnutrition
Theophylline	10-20 mg/dl	Relaxes smooth muscle of bronchi and pulmonary blood vessels	Abdominal discomfort, anorexia, dysrhythmias, nausea, vomiting, nervousness, irritability, tachycardia	Smoking and phenytoin (Dilantin) shortens half-life
Troponin I (cTnI)	<0.35 ng/ml	Serum marker for cardiac disease. Elevates within 3 hrs of AMI Remains elevated for 5-9 days More specific then troponin T	Acute MI, minor myocardial damage, unstable angina pectoris	
Troponin T (cTnT)	<0.20 ng/L	Same as cTnI Remains elevated for 10-14 days	Same as cTnI	

Test	Normal Value	Clinical Significance	Clinical Increases	Clinical Decreases
Blood Urea Nitrogen (BUN)	8-25 mg/dL SI 2.9-8.9 mmol/L (Indicator of kidney function)	End product of protein metabolism.	Adrenal or renal insufficiency, CHF, dehydration, ↓renal flow, N2 metabolism, GI bleed, shock, urine obstruction.	Hepatic failure, low protein diet, nephrosis, pregnancy

Microbiology

Test	Normal Value	Clinical Significance	Clinical Increases	Clinical Decreases
AFB Smear and Culture	No organisms seen False negative? (5,000-50,000 organisms/mL = +) No growth on myobacterial agar x 6-8 wks incub is generally neg for MTb	+ Smear = poss active case of MTb (or one of 50 other species, incl. non-mycobateria spp.)	+ Culture indicates MTb present in culture site (i.e., lungs, stomach, kidneys, GI, blood, marrow, sterile body fluids, tissue, wound aspirate)	

5-10

Urine Tests

Test	Normal Value	Clinical Significance	Clinical Increases	Clinical Decreases
Urine Output	Male 900-1800 ml/day Female 600-1600 ml/day Average = 1200 ml/day	Urine output may change acid-base balance	Diuretics, diabetes insipidus, excessive intake	Dehydration, hypovolemia, injury, kidney dysfunction, shock
Urine pH	4.5-8.0	Reflects plasma pH and acid-base balance	> 7 = bacterial infection in tract, metabolic alkalosis, $\downarrow K^+$, vegetarian diet	< 6 = metabolic acidosis, protein diet
Urine glucose	None present	If glucose present: indicates serum glucose level > 160-180 mg%	Diabetes	
Urine Ketones	1+ to 3+		Ketoacidosis, starvation, diet high in protein and low in carbohydrates	

5-11

Sputum Characteristics

Condition	Mucoid	Purulent	Mucopurulent	Hemoptysis	Currant Jelly	Rusty	Prune Juice	Blood Streaked	Pink, frothy
Viral Pneumonia	×								
Tuberculosis	×	×	×	×					
Pulmonary infarct				×					
Pulmonary edema	×								×
Pneumonia (Staphlococcal)		×							
Pneumonia (Pseudomonas)		×	×						
Pneumonia (Pneumococcal)		×				×	×		
Pneumonia (Mycoplasma)	×								
Pneumonia (Klebsiella)					×		×		
Neoplasm				×	×	×			
Lung cancer	×			×	×				
Lung abcess		×	×						
Emphysema	×			×					
Cystic Fibrosis				×					
Chronic Bronchitis	×			×					
Bronchiectasis		×		×		×			
Asthma	×			×					

Normal Sputum Characteristics

- Amount: 10–100 cc/day
- Color: Clear
- Viscocity: Thin/None
- Odor:

Type	Characteristics
Mucoid	clear, thin, frothy
Purulent	yellor or green, thick, viscid, offen, odor pus
Mucopurulent	both mucoid and purulent
Hemoptysis	bright red, frothy blood
Currant Jelly	blood clots
Rusty	mucopurulent with red tinge
Prune Juice	dark brown, mucopurulent, offensive odor
Blood Streaked	
Pink, frothy	

Sputum Collection	
Indications	To obtain sputum specimen for various laboratory testing
Contra-indications	Dependent on technique, may include: Mental Status, Age (Directed Cough), Excessive Oral Secretions, etc.
Procedure	• Explain procedure to pt • Before collection/induction, have pt blow nose and rinse out mouth • Best obtained early AM • Have pt drink extra fluids night before • Pt should sit upright when coughing • Have pt forcefully cough and spit specimen into collection cup • Do not touch edge/inside of cup • If clear/watery, probable saliva • If thick/colorful, likely good sample • Typical quantity: routine (2-3 cc), TB and fungus (10-15 cc) • Should go to lab within 1 hour • Ideal specimen is obtained by bypassing oral cavity, directly into specimen container.

Sputum Induction	
Indications	If unable to obtain sample in traditional methods, you may need to induce
Contraindications	(Relative) Patients with hx of bronchospasm, asthma, etc.
Procedure	• Brief application of 3-7% hypertonic saline (consider Ultrasonic or high-output heated jet) • After nebulizing, following the Procedure above for Collection
Hazards	• May cause bronchospasm (may administer SABA prior to hypertonic to help prevent)

Confirm Order for Sputum Culture

Preparation/Collection
(see previous page)

Least
Invasive

Consider the
Risks vs. Benefits
of each step,
going from
Least to Most
Invasive.

Consider
Hazards and
Contraindications
at each Step, as
appropriate

Directed Cough
(Huff Technique)

**Addition of
PEP Device**

**Nebulized
Normal Saline**
(0.9%),
Consider Hypertonic
with Caution

**Nasal Tracheal
Suction**

**Recommend
Bronchial
Alveolar
Lavage**

Most
Invasive

Verify Good Sample
(quantity - 2-3 mL routinely, clean container, thick, colorful)

6 PULMONARY FUNCTION TESTS

CONTENTS

!

Typical Pulmonary Function Values*

Most PFT parameters do not have a single normal value. A normal or predicted value is an interactive function of BSA, age, height, weight, sex, race, etc. Also, there are no universally accepted criteria for determining degrees of abnormality.

Lung Volumes (BTPS)		
IC	Inspiratory Capacity	3.60 L
IRV	Inspiratory Reserve Volume	3.10 L
ERV	Expiratory Reserve Volume	1.20 L
VC	Vital Capacity	4.80 L
RV	Residual Volume	1.20 L
FRC	Functional Residual Capacity	2.40 L
V_{TG}	Thoracic Gas Volume	2.40 L
TLC	Total Lung Capacity	6.00 L
RV/VC	Residual Volume/VC	33%
RV/TLC	Residual Volume/TLC	20%
Ventilation (BTPS)		
V_T ●	Tidal Volume	0.50 L
RR ●	Respiratory Rate	12/min
$\dot{V}_E$ ●	Minute Volume	6.00 L/min
V_D	Dead Space Volume	150 mL
$\dot{V}_A$	Alveolar Ventilation	4.20 L/min
V_D/V_T	Dead Space/Tidal Volume Ratio	0.30

● Indicates Values that can be Measured with Bedside Spirometry

Mechanics of Breathing

FVC ●	Forced Vital Capacity	4.80 L
SVC ●	Slow Vital Capacity	4.80 L
FIVC ●	Forced Inspiratory Vital Capacity	4.80 L
FEV$_T$ ●	Forced Exp Volume over Time	(varies)
FEV 1%	Forced Exp Volume Ratio (1 sec)	83%
FEV 3%	Forced Exp Volume Ratio (3 secs)	97%
FEF ● 200-1200	Forced Expiratory Flow from 200cc to 1200cc	400 L/min
PEF ●	Peak Expiratory Flow	600 L/min
FEF 25-75 ●	Forced Expiratory Flow from 25-75% of FVC	4.70 L/sec
FIF 25-75 (FIFmax)	Forced Inspiratory Flow from 25-75% of FIVC	5.00 L/sec
$\dot{V}$max 50	Forced Expiratory Flow at 50% of FVC	5.00 L/sec
MVV ●	Maximal Voluntary Ventilation	170 L/min
C_L	Static Compliance of Lungs	0.2 L/cm H_2O
C_{LT}	Static Compliance of Lungs and Thoracic Cage	0.1 L/cm H_2O
Raw	Airway Resistance	1.50 cmH2O/L/sec
Rpul	Pulmonary Resistance	2.00 cmH2O/L/sec
Gaw	Airway Conductance	0.66 L/sec/cmH2O
SGaw	Specific Conductance	0.22 L/sec/cmH2O/L
W rest	Work of Quiet Breathing	0.5 kg • M/min
W max	Maximal Work of Breathing	10 kg • M/breath
MIP ●	Maximal Inspiratory Pressure	- 80 mm Hg
MEP	Maximal Expiratory Pressure	120 mm Hg

Distribution of Inspired Gas

$\dot{V}_A$	Alveolar Ventilation	4.20 L/min
V_D/V_T	Physiological Deadspace Ratio	< 30
SBN$_2$	Single-Breath N$_2$ Test ΔN$_2$ from 750-1250 mL expired	< 1.5% N$_2$
7 Minute N$_2$	Alveolar N$_2$ after 7 min of O$_2$	< 2.5% N$_2$
CV	Closing Volume	400 mL
CV/VC	Closing Volume/VC Ratio	9%
CC	Closing Capacity	1600 mL
CC/TLC	Closing Capacity/TLC Ratio	32%
Slope of Phase III in Single-Breath N$_2$ Test		< 2% N$_2$/L

● Indicates Values that can be Measured with Bedside Spirometry

Pulmonary Blood Flow		
CO	Cardiac Output	5.40 L/min
$\dot{Q}_T$	Total Perfusion of the Lung	5.20 L/min
$\dot{Q}_{Sphys}$	Physiological shunt	< 7%
$\dot{Q}_{Sanat}$	Anatomic shunt	< 3%
$\dot{Q}_{Cpul}$	Pulmonary Cap. Blood Volume	75-100 mL
Alveolar Ventilation/Perfusion		
$\dot{V}_A$	Alveolar Ventilation	4.20 L/min
$\dot{Q}_{Cpul}$	Pulmonary Capillary Blood Flow	5.20 L/min
$\dot{V}_A/\dot{Q}_C$	Alveolar Ventilation/Blood Flow	0.8
Gas Exchange		
$\dot{V}_{CO_2}$	CO_2 Production	200 mL/min
$\dot{V}_{O_2}$	O_2 Consumption	250 mL/min
RQ	Respiratory Quotient ($\dot{V}_{CO_2}/\dot{V}_{O_2}$)	0.8 (tissue level)
RER	Respiratory Exchange Ratio (CO_2 output / O_2 uptake)	0.8 (end-tidal level)
Alveolar Gas		
P_{AO_2}	Partial Press of Alveolar O_2	109 mm Hg
P_{ACO_2}	Partial Press of Alveolar CO_2	40 mm Hg
Arterial Blood		
PaO_2	Partial Press of Arterial PaO_2	99 mm Hg
SaO_2	O_2 Saturation of Arterial Blood	97%
pH	Negative log of H^+ concentration	7.40
$PaCO_2$	Partial Press of Arterial CO_2	40 mm Hg
PaO_2 on 100	P.P. While Breathing 100% O_2	640 mm Hg
P_{A-aO_2}	A-aO_2 Gradient	10 mm Hg
P_{A-aO_2}	A-aO_2 Gradient on 100% O_2	33 mm Hg
CaO_2	Content of Arterial O_2	20 vol%
$C\bar{V}O_2$	Content of Mixed Venous O_2	15 vol%
$Ca-\bar{V}O_2$	A-V difference of O_2 Content	5 vol%
Diffusion		
D_{LCO}	Diffusing Capacity (Single Breath)	25/17 mL/min/mmHg
$D_L/\dot{V}_A$	Diffusing Capacity/$\dot{V}_A$ (KCO)	4
Control Of Ventilation		
Ventilatory Response to Hypercapnia		0.50 L/min/mmHg
Ventilatory Response to Hypoxia		0.20 L/min/ΔSO_2
Arterial Blood PO_2 during Moderate Excerise		95 mm Hg

* Typical values for a young male at sea level. Height 165 cm, weight 64 kg, body surface area 1.7 m^2.

Overview Of Patterns Of Abnormal Pulmonary Functions

PF Tests	Obstructive				Restrictive
	Asthma	Emphysema	Chronic Bronchitis	Small Airway Disease	
Lung Volumes					
SVC	N↓	N↓	N↓	N	↓
RV	↑	↑	↑	N↑	N↓
FRC	↑	↑	↑	N	N↓
TLC	N↑	↑	N↑	N	↓
RV/TLC	↑	↑	↑	N↑	N↑
Mechanics					
FVC	↓	↓	N↓	N	↓
FEV$_1$	↓	↓	↓	N	N
FEF 200-1200	N↓	N↓	↓	N	N↓
FEF 25-75	↓	↓	↓	↓	N↓
PEF	↓	↓	↓	N	N↓
MVV	↓	↓	↓	N	N↓
Cstat	N	↑	N	N	↓
Cdyn	↓	↓	↓	N↓	↓
Raw	↑	N↓	↑	N	N
CV	↑	↑	↑	N↑	N↑
V/Q Relationships					
A-a Gradient	↑	↑	↑	↑	N↑
$\dot{Q}_S/\dot{Q}_T$	↑	↑	↑	↑	N↑
V$_D$/V$_T$	↑	↑	↑	N↑	↑
D$_L$CO	N	↓	N	N	N↓

N = Normal, ↑ = Increased, ↓ = Decreased

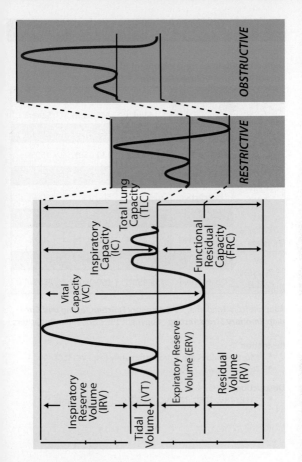

Volumes and Capacities
(see 6-1 for values)
(see 6-7 for descriptions of maneuvers)

**General Guidelines for Assignment of
Severity of Lung Volume Disorders**

Volume (Normal)	Disorder	Severity		
		Mild	Moderate	Severe
TLC (80-120% Pred)	Restrictive	70-80%	60-70%	< 60%
	Obstructive	120-130%	130-150%	> 150%
VC (> 90% Pred)	Restrictive	70-90%	50-70%	< 50%
	Obstructive	70-90%	50-70%	< 50%
FRC (65-135% Pred)	Restrictive	55-65%	45-55%	< 45%
	Obstructive	135-150%	150-200%	> 200%
RV (65-135% Pred)	Restrictive	55-65%	45-55%	< 45%
	Obstructive	135-150%	150-250%	>250%

Adapted from Madama, V., *Pulmonary Function Testing and Cardiopulmonary Stress Testing*. Copyright 1993 by Delmar Publishers.

Restriction
- Most all values are ↓ proportionately (esp. VC, TLC).
- Normal flows

Obstruction
- ↑TLC, ↑RV, ↑FRC, ↑RV/VC, ↑RV/TLC, ↓ VC, & ↓ Flows

Spirometry
Lung Volumes and Capacities

Test	Description
Tidal Volume (V$_T$)	Volume of gas moved in or out of the lungs in a normal resting breath.
Inspiratory Reserve Volume (IRV)	Maximum volume of gas inspired from end-tidal inspiration.
Inspiratory Capacity (IC)	Maximum volume of gas inspired from resting expiratory level (VT + IRV).
Expiratory Reserve Volume (ERV)	Maximum volume of gas expired from resting expiratory level.
Vital Capacity (VC)	Maximum volume of gas expired after a maximum inspiration (IC + ERV).
Residual Volume (RV)	Volume of gas in the lungs at the end of a maximum expiration.
Total Lung Capacity (TLC)	Volume of gas in lungs at the end of a maximum inspiration.
RV/TLC	Residual volume expressed as a percent of total lung capacity.
Functional Residual Capacity (FRC)	Volume in lungs at resting expiratory level (ERV + RV).
Thoracic Gas Volume (V$_{TG}$)	Volume of gas in entire thoracic cavity at resting expiratory level whether or not it communicates with the airways.

Normal Values
- Normal values may vary within 20% of predicted.
- Values will change with position, age, sex, height, altitude, race/ethnicity.

Other Tests for Measuring Lung Volumes
- Helium (He) Dilution: Measures RV + FRC
- Nitrogen (N2) Washout: Measures RV + FRC
- Body Plethysmography: Measures V$_{TG}$ (FRC) + Raw

PULMONARY MECHANICS

Test	Description	Interpretation
Slow Vital Capacity (SVC)	Maximum volume of gas exhaled slowly after a maximum inspiration.	Both SVC and FVC are effort dependent. SVC should = FVC.
Forced Vital Capacity (FVC)	Maximum volume of gas exhaled forcefully after a maximum inspiration.	Restrictive: ↓SVC & ↓FVC; Obstructive: SVC may be normal, ↓FVC > ↓SVC
Forced Expiratory Volume, timed (FEVt)	A volume of gas measured at a specific time interval during an FVC maneuver.	<table><tr><td>Time</td><td>%</td><td>Normal</td><td>Obstructive</td><td>Restrictive</td></tr><tr><td>0.5</td><td>60</td><td></td><td></td><td></td></tr><tr><td>1.0</td><td>83</td><td>>70%</td><td><70%</td><td>>70% usually</td></tr><tr><td>2.0</td><td>94</td><td></td><td></td><td></td></tr><tr><td>3.0</td><td>97</td><td>>95%</td><td><95%</td><td>>95%</td></tr></table>
Forced Expiratory Volume, percent (FEVt%, FEVt/FVC)	The percent of gas forcefully exhaled during an FVC maneuver.	
Forced Expiratory Flow 25-75% (FEF25-75, MMEF, MMF)	Average forced expiratory flow during the middle half of an FVC (mid-maximal expiratory flow)	Measures average flow through smaller airways. Normal = 4.7 L/sec (282 L/min). ↓ in early stages of obstructive. Normal in restrictive.
Forced Expiratory Flow 200-1200 (FEF200-1200, MEF)	Average forced expiratory flow of one liter of gas after the first 200 mL is exhaled during an FVC (maximal expiratory flow).	Measures average flow through larger airways. Normal = 6-7 L/sec (400 L/min). ↓ = mechanical problem or severe obstruction. Effort dependent.
Peak Expiratory Flow (PEF, FEFmax)	Maximum instantaneous flow attained during an FVC maneuver.	Indication of ability to cough. Normal = 10 L/sec (600 L/min)

6-8

Peak Inspiratory Flow (PIF)	Maximum instantaneous flow attained during a forceful inspiration. (Very effort dependent). Normal = 5 L/sec (300 L/min). PIF > PEF in obstruction, PIF = PEF in restriction.
Maximum Voluntary Ventilation (MVV, MBC)	Total volume of gas a subject can breathe in and out with maximum effort in one minute (maximum breathing capacity). Indicates efficiency of total pulmonary system: muscles, compliance, resistance, neurological coordination. Very effort dependent. ↓ with moderate obstruction (exaggerates air-trapping) and severe restriction.

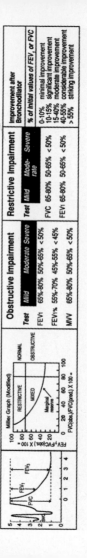

Obstructive Impairment

Test	Mild	Moderate	Severe
FEV₁	65%-80%	50%-65%	<50%
FEV₁%	55%-70%	45%-55%	<45%
MVV	65%-80%	50%-65%	<50%

Restrictive Impairment

Test	Mild	Moderate	Severe
FVC	65-80%	50-65%	<50%
FEV₁	65-80%	50-65%	<50%

Improvement after Bronchodilator

% of initial values of FEV, or FVC	
0-10%	minimal improvement
10-15%	significant improvement
15-40%	moderate improvement
40-55%	considerable improvement
>55%	striking improvement

6-9

COMPLIANCE AND RESISTANCE

Test	Description	Interpretation
Static Compliance (Cstat) 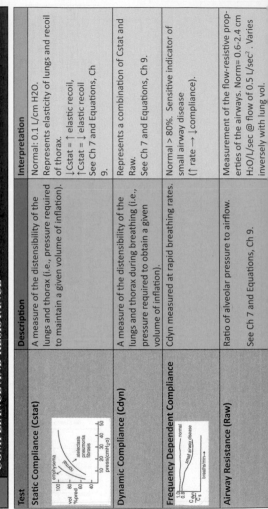	A measure of the distensibility of the lungs and thorax (i.e., pressure required to maintain a given volume of inflation).	Normal: 0.1 L/cm H2O. Represents elasticity of lungs and recoil of thorax. ↓Cstat = ↑ elastic recoil ↑Cstat = ↓ elastic recoil See Ch 7 and Equations, Ch 9.
Dynamic Compliance (Cdyn)	A measure of the distensibility of the lungs and thorax during breathing (i.e., pressure required to obtain a given volume of inflation).	Represents a combination of Cstat and Raw. See Ch 7 and Equations, Ch 9.
Frequency Dependent Compliance	Cdyn measured at rapid breathing rates.	Normal > 80%. Sensitive indicator of small airway disease (↑ rate → ↓ compliance).
Airway Resistance (Raw)	Ratio of alveolar pressure to airflow. See Ch 7 and Equations, Ch 9.	Measurement of the flow-resistive properties of the airways. Norm= 0.6-2.4 cm H2O/L/sec @ flow of 0.5 L/sec². Varies inversely with lung vol.

Test		Description	Interpretation
Flow Volume Loop (Curve) (MEF + MIF)		Test of flow and volume relationships during maximal inspiratory and expiratory maneuvers. $\dot{V}$max 75 = max flow at 75 % of FVC (50 = 50%, 25 = 25%)	Test of small airway disease. Shapes of curves are qualitative diagnostic tests. Flow at lower 2/3 volume becomes less effort-dependent. $\dot{V}$max provides a quantitative value of flow.
	$\Delta\dot{V}$max 50	Difference in $\Delta\dot{V}$50 when using two gases of differing densities.	Less dense gas = ↓ resistance at ↑ lung volumes, where airflow is turbulent. Laminar flow predominates at lower lung volumes where resistance is independent of gas density. The lung volume at which the gas density begins to effect is called the **Viso $\dot{V}$**. Small airway disease with ↑resistance causes site of flow limitation to occur at ↑ volumes.
	Viso $\dot{V}$	Volume of lungs at which flows become identical using two gases of different density (i.e., flow independent of density)	

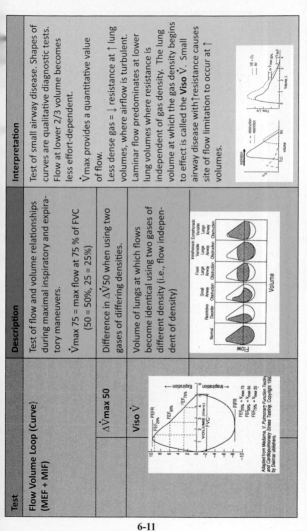

Adapted from Madama, V. *Pulmonary Function Testing and Cardiopulmonary Stress Testing* Copyright 1993 by Delmar Publishers.

6-11

GAS DISTRIBUTION TESTS

Test	Description	Interpretation
Single Breath Nitrogen Washout (SBN$_2$) or Single Breath O$_2$ Test (SBO$_2$) (ΔN$_2$ 750-1250)	Rise in N$_2$ in 500 mL of exhaled gas after exhalation of the first 750 mL following inhalation of 100% O$_2$.	Index of evenness of ventilation. Normal (even) ventilation = rise of N$_2$ % along Phase 3 < 1.5%. > 1.5% = uneven distribution and/or uneven expiratory flow. (See next pg)
Closing Volume (CV)	Volume of gas expired between onset of airway closure (Phase 4) and RV. Expressed as % of FVC. Normal < 10%. ↑CV = early obstruction, age, CHF, restriction when FRC < CV. Sensitive test to measure point of small airway closure. Used to determine evenness of ventilation. Basilar airways close first (↓O2). Remainder of exhaled air is from apical airways (↑N2).	
Closing Capacity (CC)	Closing volume plus RV. Expressed as % of TLC.	CC = measurement of choice because it includes the ↑RV in obstructive disorders. Normal < 32%. ↑ CV/VC and CC/TLC = obstructive
Nitrogen Washout Test (7 minute)	Concentration of N$_2$ remaining in alveolar gas after 7 minutes of breathing 100% O$_2$.	Washout curve is indicative of distribution of ventilation. Normal = < 2.5% (See next pg)
Radioxenon Lung Scan (133Xe)	Radiographic scan of lung using radioisotope 133 Xe	Determines how rapidly and how even the gas is distributed. Washing out shows areas of ↑ ventilation and/or trapped gas.

Nitrogen Washout Test

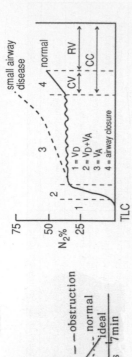

Single Breath Nitrogen Washout Test (SBN2)

Dead Space Ratio (V_D/V_T)	Ratio of volume of gas not participating in gas exchange in a normal breath compared to total volume of the breath.	Normal < 0.3 (1 mL/lb IBW). Estimate of functional lung capacity and indication of V/Q equality. ↑ ratio = ↑ V_D = ↑ wasted ventilation. See Ch 9
Alveolar Ventilation ($\dot{V}_A$)	Volume of gas /unit time (L/min) participating in gas exchange.	Normal = 4-5 L/min with wide variation. Calculation less accurate as V/Q inequality increases. See Ch 9

6-13

BLOOD FLOW DISTRIBUTION

Test	Description	Interpretation
Single Breath CO_2 Elimination	Measurement of CO_2 concentration during exhalation.	Index of uniformity of ventilation to blood flow. Uneven V/Q → different lung areas and different emptying rates → linear curve.
Clinical Shunt ($\dot{Q}s/\dot{Q}t$)	Quantitative measurement of fraction of blood passing by the lungs and not participating in gas exchange.	Normal = 3-5%. ↑shunt = ↑ amount of mixed venous blood not coming in contact with alveolar air. See Equations, Ch 9.
Radioxenon Elimination (133Xe)	Qualitative view of Xe diffusing from the blood into the lungs.	Analysis of V/Q equality.
Angiogram	Roetgenogram view of the pulmonary vessels	Qualitative analysis of lung perfusion.
Lung Perfusion Scan	Photoscintography of lung perfusion	

DIFFUSION CAPACITY

Single Breath or Steady State (DLCO_SB or SS)	Tests to measure all factors affecting diffusion across A-C membrane. Normal = 25 mL CO/min/mm Hg.	DLCO is also directly related to alveolar volume. Normal DLCO/V̇A = 4 (20 mL/min/mm Hg/5L). ↓ DLCO (due to ↓ V̇A) = restriction ↓ DLCO (due to V/Q mismatch; uneven inspired volume/alveolar volume) = obstruction.

Reference equations vary widely, particularly for DLCO where often cited values are based upon people who have never smoked with various age-ranges. *

It is advisable, therefore, to review PFT results in context of the patient's quality-of-life.

* from Miller & Enright. PFT Interpretive Strategies: American Thoracic Society/ European Respiratory Society 2005 Guideline Gaps. Respiratory Care, Volume 57, Issue 1, 2012.

Simplified Algorithm for Assessing Lung Function*

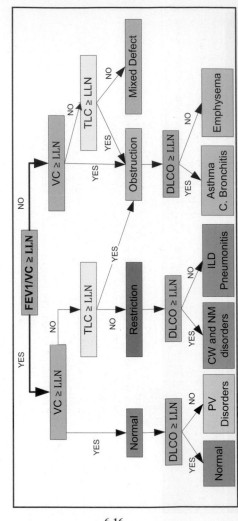

LLN: lower limits of normal; PV: pulmonary vascular; CW: chest wall; NM: neuromuscular; ILD: interstitial lung disease

Reprinted with permission[1]. See notes and explanations on the next page.

6-16

*Note:
Two LLNs are currently in use.

1. LLN % - Many PFT labs still use LLN%
(i.e., 80% of the predicted value for FEV1 and FVC; and 70% of the
predicted value for FEV1/FVC ratio). The use of a fixed percentage
completely ignores changes in predicted values due to age, height,
sex, and race/ethnic group, and can lead to important errors in interpreting lung function, and is therefore, no longer recommended.

The ATS/ERS Statement on COPD and GOLD COPD Standards
defines COPD as a post-bronchodilator FEV1/FVC ratio < 0.7. This is
an oversimplification and approximation meant for initial screening
purposes only, and is not meant to be applied in the PFT lab as the
true LLN for all populations.

2. LLN CI - In the USA, the more valid and currently recommended
approach by the ATS/ERS Pulmonary Function Testing Guidelines,
is to define the LLN as the lower fifth percentile, or 95% confidence
limit, of the predicted value (LLN CI), (i.e., the value exceeded by
95% of normal individuals of the same gender, age, height, and
race/ethnic group).

ATS/ERS also recommends adoption of the NHANES III (National
Health and Nutrition Examination Survey) reference equations for
adults, for predicted normals.

---

1. ATS/ERS Task Force: Standardization of Lung Function Testing,
Series #5; Pellegrino, R., et al., Interpretative strategies for lung
function tests. The European Respiratory Journal , 26 (5), 948-968,
2005.

2. Aggarwal, A., et al., Comparison of fixed percentage method and
lower confidence limits for defining limits of normality for interpretation of spirometry. Respiratory Care , Vol 51, #7, 2006.

Evidence-Based Guidelines

- ATS/ERS Standardization of Lung Function Testing: General Considerations for Lung Function Testing
- ATS/ERS Standardization of Lung Function Testing: Standardization of the Measurement of Lung Volumes
- ATS/ERS Standardization of the Single Breath Determination of Carbon Monoxide Uptake in the Lung
- ATS Statement: Guidelines for the Six-Minute Walk Test
- ATS Guidelines for Methacoline and Exercise Challenge Testing

AARC Clinical Practice Guidelines:

- Body Plethysmography 2001 Revision & Update
- Infant/Toddler Pulmonary Function Tests—2008 Revision & Update
- Metabolic Measurement using Indirect Calorimetry during Mechanical Ventilation 2004 Revision & Update
- Methacholine Challenge Testing 2001 Revision & Update
- Single-Breath Carbon Monoxide Diffusing Capacity 1999 Revision & Update
- Spirometry 1996 Revision & Update
- Static Lung Volumes 2001 Revision & Update

7 PULMONARY DYNAMICS

CONTENTS

MECHANICS OF VENTILATION

Volume & Pressure Changes During Spont. Breathing

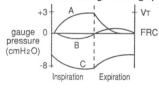

A: Lung Volume
B: Alveolar Pressure
C: Intrathoracic Pressure

Inspiration	Diaphragm/chest muscles contract → ↑intrathoracic vol. → ↓ intrathoracic (pleural) pressure + pleural cohesion → ↑ intrapulmonary (lung) vol → ↓ intrapulmonary (alveoli) pressure → air moves down gradient (in).
Active	
Expiration	Muscles relax, plus elastic recoil of lung → ↓ intrapulmonary vol- ume → ↑intrapulmonary press → air moves down gradient (out).
Passive	

Pressures and Pressure Gradients

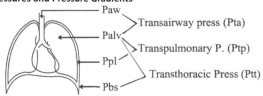

Paw
Palv — Transairway press (Pta)
Ppl — Transpulmonary P. (Ptp)
Pbs — Transthoracic Press (Ptt)

Pressures*

Abbreviation	Definition	Also Known As	
Paw, Pawo, or Pm	Pressure at airway (opening or mouth)	Mouth pressure	Normally atmospheric (zero), unless positive airway pressure is applied
Palv	Pressure in the alveoli	Intrapulmonary pressure, alveoli pressure (Pₐ)	Varies during breathing cycle
Ppl	Pressure in pleural space	Intrapleural pressure (Pᵢₚ) or intrathoracic pressure (Pᵢₜ)	Varies during breathing cycle. Normally negative during quiet spontaneous breathing
Patm or Pbs	Pressure at body surface	Atmospheric (barometric) pressure (Pв)	Normally zero, unless negative pressure is applied

Pressure Gradients

Pta	Transairway pressure gradient, Pta = Paw - Palv	Pressure difference down the airway.	Responsible for gas flow into and out of the lungs.
Ptp	Transpulmonary pressure gradient, Ptp = Palv - Ppl	Pressure difference across the lung.	Responsible for degree of and maintenance of alveolar inflation or volume change.
Ptt	Transthoracic pressure gradient, Ptt = Patm- Palv	Pressure difference across the lung and chest wall.	Total pressure necessary to expand or contract the lungs and chest wall together.

Clinical Note: Transrespiratory pressure gradient = Paw – Pbs.

Transmural pressure gradient (Ptm) = Pressure gradient across a vessel wall (intravascular pressure [Pᵢᵥ] minus Pᵢₜ).

* Pressures are measured as gauge pressure in cm H2O and expressed relative to atmospheric pressure. Hence, a pressure of 5 cm H2O is atmospheric (1034 cm H2O) plus 5 cm H2O.

(See Chapter 9 for clinical equations)

Compliance = ease of distention
= 1/difficulty of distention (static impedance)
= 1/elastance
= 1/elastic forces + surface tension

↑ Elastance = ↓ Compliance	↓ Elastance = ↑ Compliance

Static Compliance (Cstat)	Total compliance of lung and thorax $C_{LT} = \Delta V/\Delta P$
Dynamic Compliance (Cdyn)	Total impendance Cdyn = Cstat = Raw
Airway Resistance (Raw)	Impedance to Airflow Raw = ΔP/flow = 0.6 - 2.4 cmH2O/L/sec @ 0.5 L/sec (norm)
Time Constant (TC)	Filling or Emptying Time of the Lung (Cstat x Raw) - See Chapter 9

Time Constant Examples	Normal Lung Unit	TC = 0.1 L/cmH2O x 2.0 cmH2O/L/Sec = (0.1) x (4.0) = 0.2 sec
	Asthma	TC = 0.1 L/cmH2O x 4.0 cmH2O/L/Sec = (0.1) x (2.0) = 0.4 sec
	Fibrosis	TC = 0.05 L/cmH20 x 2.0 H2O/L/Sec = (0.05) x (2.0) = 0.1 sec

SEE FIGURE NEXT PAGE

!

A **Long Time Constant** results in alveoli that fill slowly on inspiration (so take even longer to empty)

A **Short Time Constant** results in alveoli that fill and empty quickly

Expiratory Airway Resistance is usually higher than Inspiratory Resistance.

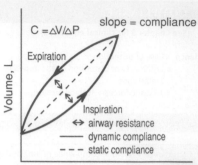

$C = \Delta V/\Delta P$ slope = compliance

Expiration

Volume, L

Inspiration
↔ airway resistance
— dynamic compliance
--- static compliance

Transpulmonary pressure, cmH$_2$O

DISTRIBUTION OF VENTILATION

Minute Ventilation ($\dot{V}_E$)	Total air moved in or out of the lungs in one minute (V_T x f) ($\dot{V}_A + \dot{V}_D$)
Alveolar Ventilation ($\dot{V}_A$)	Ventilation which participates in gas exchange (V_A x f) ($\dot{V}_E - \dot{V}_D$)
Deadspace Ventilation ($\dot{V}_D$)	Ventilation which does not participate in gas exchange (V_D x f) ($\dot{V}_E - \dot{V}_A$)

Types of Deadspace

VDphys	=	VDanat	+	VDalv	+	VDmech
Physiological (Total)	=	*Anatomical* Conducting passages, 1/3 V_T or 1cc/lb IBW, ↓ ½ with trach	+	Alveolar Alveoli without perfusion	+	Mechanical Air in tubing that is rebreathed.

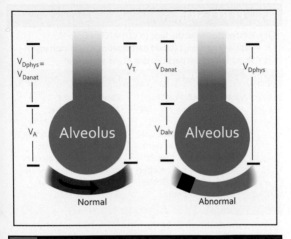

$V_{Dphys} = V_{Danat}$

V_A

V_T

V_{Danat}

V_{Dalv}

V_{Dphys}

Alveolus

Alveolus

Normal

Abnormal

Distribution of Vent. through Lung Regions

Spontaneous Ventilation: Air moving into the lungs at FRC will go to the gravity-dependent areas. Near TLC distribution will be more even.

Mechanical Ventilation (Positive Pressure): Air will take the path of least resistance, usually the uppermost areas. This is why large tidal volumes (10-15 cc/kg PBW) *were* sometimes given - so that air will fill the uppermost portions and then move into the gravity dependent portions where most of the perfusion is.

> **!**
> While large tidal volumes may distribute physiologically, it is important to remember that lung units are often not "homogenous" (one single unit). Because of this, current evidence-based medicine supports delivered tidal volumes in the 6-8 cc/kg PBW range (or less). The goal is to protect healthy lung units which are often more compliant - air will follow the path of least resistance.

$\dot{Q}_T$ = Total perfusion of the lung ($\approx$ CO) = ($\dot{Q}_c + \dot{Q}_s$)
$\dot{Q}_c$ = Capillary perfusion (blood participating in gas exchange)
$\dot{Q}_s$ = Shunt (blood not participating in gas exchange)

$\dot{Q}_{sphys}$ =	$\dot{Q}_{sanat}$ +	$\dot{Q}_{scap}$
Physiological Shunt (Total)	Anatomical Shunt Universal = 2 - 5% CO. Pleural, thebesian, & bronchial veins, congenital heart defects, AV malformations, vascular lung tumors.	Capillary Shunt Alveolar collapse, pneumothorax, airway obstruction, ↓surfactant, atelectasis, space occupying lesions, alveolar filling (secretions, edema, abscess, pneumonia), diffusion defect.

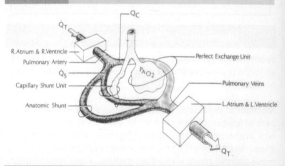

Perfusion Zones

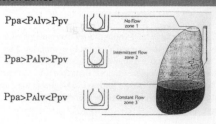

Ppa<PAlv>Ppv		No Flow zone 1
Ppa>PAlv>Ppv		Intermittent flow zone 2
Ppa>PAlv<Ppv		Constant Flow zone 3

Zone levels are dependent on cardiac output, alveolar pressure (vol, esp. PEEP), and gravity. Most blood flow occurs in zone 3, which will be the gravity dependent areas.

Body position has a significant effect on the distribution of pulmonary blood flow, as shown in the erect (A), supine (lying on the back) (B), and lateral (lying on the side) (C), positions.

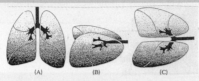

(A)   (B)   (C)

Above figures reprinted with permission from Shapiro, B, et.al.: Clinical Application of Arterial Blood Gases, 3rd Ed., Yearbook Publishers, 1982.

VENTILATION/PERFUSION ($\dot{V}/\dot{Q}$)

Normal Lung = $\dot{V}/\dot{Q}$ = 4L/min / 5L/min = 0.8 (normal ratio)

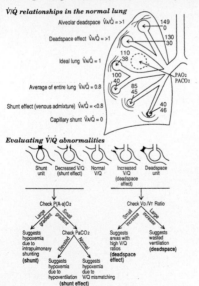

Adapted from Harper, R.W.: A Guide to Respiratory Care: Phys. & Clin. Applic. Copyright 1981: by J.B. Lippincott Co., Philadelphia.

7-7

Additional Resources

West, John, MD. 8th Ed., 2008. Respiratory Physiology: the Essentials

See Oakes' **RespiratoryUpdate.com** for further information and explanations of Pulmonary Dynamics, including direct links to:

- Lung Dynamics
- Ventilation-Perfusion Relationships
- O2 and CO2 Transport and Diffusion,

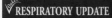

RESPIRATORY UPDATE

THE Virtual Critical Care Library

8 CARDIOVASCULAR DYNAMICS

CONTENTS

HEMODYNAMIC PARAMETERS

Measured		Abbreviation	Normal Value
Arterial Blood Pressure	Systolic	BPsys	100-140 mmHg
	Mean	$\overline{BP}$ or MAP	70-105 mmHg
	Diastolic	BPdia	60-80 mmHg
	Pulse Pressure	PP	20-80 mmHg
Cardiac Output		CO	4-8 L/min
Central Venous Pressure		CVP	0-6 mmHg 0-8 cmH20
Heart Rate		HR	60-100 beats/min
Pulmonary Artery Pressures (PAP)	Systolic	PASP	15-25 mmHg
	Mean	PAMP or $\overline{PAP}$	10-15 mmHg
	Diastolic	PADP	8-15 mmHg
	End Diastolic	PAEDP	0-12 mmHg
	Wedge	PAWP	4-12 mmHg
Right Atrial Pressure		RAP or $\overline{RAP}$	0-6 mmHg
Right Ventricular End Diastolic Pressure		RVEDP	0-5 mmHg
Right Ventricular End Systolic Pressure		RVESP	15-25 mmHg

Derived	Abbrev	Normal Value
Body Surface Area	BSA	See chapter 9
Cardiac Index	CI	2.5-4.4 L/min/m^2
Left Atrial Pressure	LAP	4-12 mmHg
Left Ventricular End Diastolic Pressure	LVEDP	4-12 mmHg
Left Ventricular End Systolic Pressure	LVESP	100-140 mmHg
Left Ventricular Stroke Work	LVSW	60-80 gm/m/beat
Left Ventricular Stroke Work Index	LVSWI	40-75 gm/m/beat/m^2
Pulmonary Vascular Resistance	PVR	20-200 dynes•sec•cm^{-5} 0.25-2.5 units (mmHg/L/min)
Pulmonary Vascular Resistance Index	PVRI	30-350 dynes•sec•cm^{-5}/m^2
Right Ventricular Stroke Work	RVSW	10-15 gm/m/beat
Right Ventricular Stroke Work Index	RVSWI	4-12 gm/m/beat/m^2
Stroke Volume	SV	60-120 mL/beat
Stroke Volume Index	SVI	35-75 mL/beat/m^2
Systemic Vascular Resistance	SVR	800-1600 dynes•sec•cm^{-5} 10-20 units (mmHg/L/min)
Systemic Vascular Resistance Index	SVRI	1400-2600 dynes•sec•cm^{-5}/m^2

OTHER HEMODYNAMIC PARAMETERS

Non-Invasive	Invasive			
Measured	Measured		Derived	
Capillary Refill	$PaCO_2$	PvO_2	$PA\text{-}aO_2$	$\dot{D}O_2$
$PtcCO_2$	PaO_2	$P\overline{v}O_2$	$Pa\text{-}vO_2$	LV Fx Curve
$PtcO_2$	pH	SaO_2	$Pa\text{-}\overline{v}O_2$	$M\dot{D}O_2$
SaO_2 (SpO_2)	$PvCO_2$	SvO_2	CaO_2	$M\dot{V}O_2$
Skin color/dryness	$P\overline{v}CO_2$	$S\overline{v}O_2$	$Ca\text{-}\overline{v}O_2$	O_2ER
Temp (core/skin)			CvO_2	$\dot{Q}S/\dot{Q}T$
UO			$C\overline{v}O_2$	$\dot{V}O_2$

See Chapter 9 for equations and their significance.

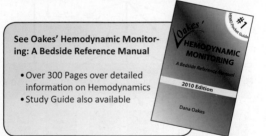

See Oakes' Hemodynamic Monitoring: A Bedside Reference Manual

• Over 300 Pages over detailed information on Hemodynamics
• Study Guide also available

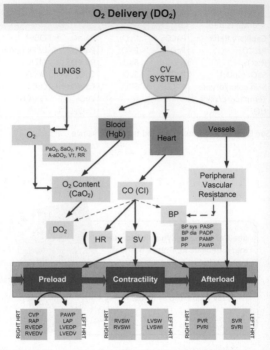

Reprinted with permission from Oakes, D.; *Hemodynamic Monitoring: A Bedside Reference Manual*. Copyright 2010 by Health Educator Publications, Inc.

OVERVIEW OF O₂ DELIVERY EQUATIONS

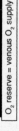

→ A - a DO₂ = PaO₂ - PaO₂

Arterial O₂ supply = O₂ delivery ($\dot{D}O_2$) (O₂ transport)

$\dot{D}O_2$ = Content arterial O₂ x cardiac output

= CaO₂ x CO x 10

normal $\dot{D}O_2$ = 1000 ml/min

O₂ extraction ratio (O₂ ER) = $\dfrac{\text{O}_2 \text{ consumption (demand)}}{\text{O}_2 \text{ delivery (supply)}}$

$O_2 ER = \dfrac{\dot{V}O_2}{\dot{D}O_2} \times 100$

Normal O₂ER = 25%

O₂ reserve = venous O₂ supply

O₂ reserve = $\dot{D}O_2 - \dot{V}O_2$

= content mixed venous
O₂ x cardiac output

= C$\bar{v}$O₂ x CO x 10

Normal O₂ reserve = 750 ml/min

Ca - $\bar{v}$O₂ = a - $\bar{v}$DO₂ = CaO₂ - C$\bar{v}$O₂

O₂ consumption ($\dot{V}O_2$) (O₂ demand)

$\dot{V}O_2$ = Fick equation

= arterial O₂ supply - venous reserve

= (CaO₂ x CO) - (C$\bar{v}$O₂ x CO) x 10

= Ca - $\bar{v}$O₂ x CO x 10

normal $\dot{V}O_2$ = 250 ml/min

Reprinted with permission from Oakes, D.; *Hemodynamic Monitoring: A Bedside Reference Manual.* Copyright 1995 by Health Educator Publications, Inc.

8-5

Blood Flow through the Heart

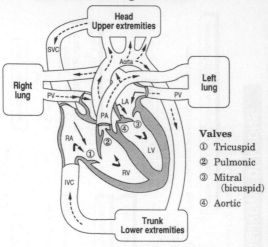

Valves
1. Tricuspid
2. Pulmonic
3. Mitral (bicuspid)
4. Aortic

Factors Controlling Blood Pressure

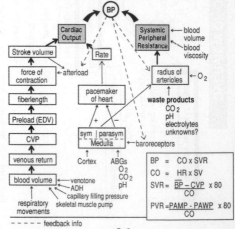

$$BP = CO \times SVR$$

$$CO = HR \times SV$$

$$SVR = \frac{\overline{BP} - CVP}{CO} \times 80$$

$$PVR = \frac{PAMP - PAWP}{CO} \times 80$$

--- feedback info

8-6

Overview of Cardiopulmonary Pressure Dynamics

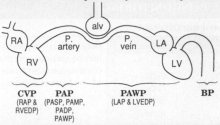

CVP	PAP	PAWP	BP
(RAP & RVEDP)	(PASP, PAMP, PADP, PAWP)	(LAP & LVEDP)	

A-Line Monitoring

Arterial Pressures

BPsys	120 mmHg
BPdia	80 mmHg
$\overline{BP}$ (MAP)	93 mmHg
PP	40 mmHg

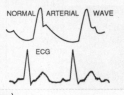

Arterial Waveform

(see page 8-1 for normal ranges)
(See page 8-9 to 8-10 for some disease-causing variations)

CVP Monitoring

Venous Pressure

CVP	0-6 mmHg
	0-8 cmH$_2$O

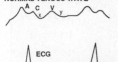

CVP Waveform

(See page 8-9 to 8-10 for some disease-causing variations)

See Oakes' Hemodynamic Monitoring: A Bedside Reference Manual

- Indications, Insertion Sites, Equipment, Techniques, Maintenance, Infection Control, Samples, Pressure and Waveform Variations, Complications, Troubleshooting, and removal of Lines

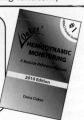

Measurements Obtainable:

Measured	Derived	Note: All invasive parameters may be obtained with the combination of an A-Line and a PA line (thermodiulution)
CO	CI	
CVP	CvO_2	
HR	$C\bar{v}O_2$	
PADP	LV (function, curve)	**A-Line**
PASP		**+**
PAWP (LAP, LVEDP)	LVSW	**PA Line parameters**
	LVSWI	**Derived**
pHv	PAMP	
$pH\bar{v}$	PVR	$a\text{-}vDO_2$ $\quad$ $M\dot{D}O_2$
$PvCO_2$	PVRI	$a\text{-}\bar{v}DO_2$ $\quad$ $M\bar{V}O_2$
$P\bar{v}CO_2$	RVSW	$Ca\text{-}vO_2$ $\quad$ O_2ER
PvO_2	RVSWI	$Ca\text{-}\bar{v}O_2$ $\quad$ $\dot{Q}s/\dot{Q}T$
$P\bar{v}O_2$	SV	CPP $\quad$ SVR
RAP (RVEDP)	SVI	$\dot{D}O_2$ $\quad$ SVRI
SvO_2	SW	$\quad$ VO_2
$S\bar{v}O_2$	SWI	

Pressures*		Waveforms
CVP	0-6 mmHg	PULMONARY ARTERY: SYSTOLIC 15-25 mmHg DIASTOLIC 8-15 mmHg MEAN 10-15 mmHg
RVSP	15-25 mmHg	
RVEDP	0-6 mmHg	
PASP	15-25 mmHg	
PADP	8-15 mmHg	
PAMP	10-15 mmHg	
PAWP	4-12 mmHg	PULMONARY WEDGE MEAN 4-12 mmHg
PADP-PAWP gradient	0-6 mmHg	

* All pressures should be measured at end-expiration (see page 8-9 and 8-10 for some disease-causing variations.

Some Disease Entities Causing PRESSURE Changes

BP	CVP	PAP	PCWP
Increased ↑P-reload: Aortic Insufficiency Arteriosclerosis Drugs (inotropes, vasopressors) Essential Hypertension	**Increased** ↑P-reload: Hypervolemia Tricuspid Insufficiency VSD ↑Afterload: ARDS COPD Chronic LVF Cor Pulmonale Hypoxemia	**Increased** Cardiac Tamponade Hypervolemia L-R shunt (ASD, VSD) LVF (CHF, MI, shock) Mitral stenosis/regurgitation ↑ PVR: Acidosis, embolism, hypertension, hypoxemia, vasopressors	**Increased** Cardiac Tamponade Constrictive Pericarditis Hypervolemia LVF (CHF, MI, shock) Mitral stenosis/regurgitation MV (esp. with PEEP) Pneumothorax
	↓ **Contractility:** Cardiac Tamponade Cardiomyopathy Constrictive Pericarditis LVF (CHF, MI, shock) MI (esp. RH) RVF		
Decreased Aortic Stenosis Arrhythmias Cardiac Tamponade LVF (CHF, MI, shock) Mitral Stenosis Shock	**Decreased** Hypovolemia: Absolute (loss) Relative (shock, drugs) MV esp. with PEEP Pulmonic Stenosis PVR ↑ (emboli, hypertension) Tricuspid Stenosis	**Decreased** Hypovolemia: Absolute (loss) Relative (shock, drugs)	**Decreased** Hypovolemia: Absolute (loss) Relative (shock, drugs)

8-9

Some Disease Entities Causing WAVEFORM Changes

BP Waveform	CVP Waveform	PAP Waveform	PAWP Waveform
Anemia	Acute RV infarct	MV (esp. with PEEP)	Acute LV infarct
Aortic stenosis/regurgitation	Arrhythmias	Note: Most variations are due to technical causes.	Arrhythmias
Arrhythmias	A-V Disassociation		Aortic Stenosis
Arteriosclerosis	Cardiac Tamponade		Cardiac Tamponade
Asthma (severe)	Constrictive Pericarditis		Constrictive Pericarditis
Cardiac Tamponade	Hypervolemia		Hypervolemia
Cardiomyopathy	Pulmonary Hypertension		LVF
Constrictive Pericarditis	Pulmonary Stenosis		Mitral stenosis/regurgitation
COPD	RVF		MV (esp. with PEEP)
Essential Hypertension	Tricuspid stenosis/regurgitation		
Hyperthyroidism			Note: Many technical causes.
Hypovolemia			
LVF			
Mitral Regurgitation			
Pulmonary Embolism			
Shock			
Systemic Hypertension			

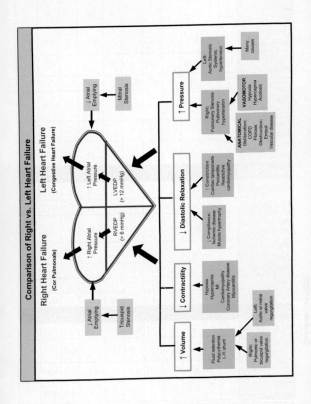

Comparison of Right vs. Left Heart Failure

Right Heart Failure
(Cor Pulmonale)

Left Heart Failure
(Congestive Heart Failure)

↓ Atrial Emptying ← Mitral Stenosis

↑ Left Atrial Pressure
LVEDP (> 12 mmHg)

↓ Atrial Emptying ← Tricuspid Stenosis

↑ Right Atrial Pressure
RVEDP (> 6 mmHg)

↑ Pressure

Left: Aortic Stenosis Systemic hypertension ← Many causes

Right: Pulmonary Stenosis Pulmonary hypertension

VASOMOTOR
Hypoxia
Hypercapnia
Acidosis

ANATOMICAL
Obliteration:
COPD
Fibrosis
Obstruction:
Emboli
Vascular disease

↓ Diastolic Relaxation

↑ Constriction
Cardiac tamponade
Pericarditis
Restrictive
cardiomyopathy

↓ Compliance:
Ischemic disease
Muscle hypertrophy

↓ Contractility

Hypoxia
Hypercapnia
M
Cardiomyopathy
Coronary Artery disease
Myocarditis

↑ Volume

Fluid retention
Polycythemia
L-R shunt

Left:
Aortic or mitral
regurgitation

Right:
Pulmonic or
tricuspid valve
regurgitation

8-11

Overview of Hemodynamic Presentation in Various Disease Entities

Disease/ Disorder	Note: Considerable Variation May Exist										
	RR	HR	BP	PP	CO	CVP	PAP	PAWP	SVR	VR	SvO₂
ARDS	↑	↑	↑↓	↑↓	N	N	↑	N	N	↑	↓
Cardiac Failure LHF	↑	↑	↑↓	↓	↓	N/↑	↑	↑	↑	↑	↓
RHF	↑	↑	↑↓	↓	↓	N	N	N	↑	N	↓
Cardiac Tamponade	↑	↑	N/↓	↓	N/↓	↑	↑	↑	↑	N/↑	N/↓
Cardiomyo-pathy	↑	↑	N/↑	↓	N/↓	↑	↑	↑	↑	N/↑	N/↓
COPD	↑	↑	N	N	N/↓	N/↑	↑	N	N/↓	↑	↓
Myocardial infarction	N/↑	↑	↑↓	↓	N/↑	N/↑	N/↑	N/↑	↑↓	N/↑	N/↓
Pulmonary edema	↑	↑	↑	N/↓	N	N	↑	↑	↑	↑	↓
Pulmonary embolism	↑	↑	N	N	N	↑	↑	N	N	↑	N/↓
Shock:											
Anaphylactic	↑	↑	↓	↓	↓	↓	↓	↓	↓	N/↑	↓
Cardiogenic	↑	↑	↓	↓	↓	N	↑↓	↑↓	N/↑	N/↑	↓
Hypovolemic compensated	↑	↑	N/↑	N/↓	↑↓	↑↓	↑↓	↑↓	↑	↓	↓
Decompen-sated	↑	↑	↓	↓	↓	↓	↓	↓	↑	↑	↓
Neurogenic	↑↓	↓	↓	↓	N/↓	↓	↓	↓	↓	↓	↓
Septic (Warm)	↑	↑	N/↓	↑	N/↑	↓	↑↓	↑↓	↓	N/↑	↑↓
Septic (Cold)	↑	↑	↓	↓	↓	↑	↑↓	↑↓	↑↓	N/↑	↑↓
Valvular:											
Aortic stenosis	↑	↑	↓	↓	↓	N/↑	↑	↑	↑	↑	↓
Aortic regurgitation	↑	↑	↓	↓	↓	↑	↑	↑	N/↑	↑	↓
Mitral stenosis	N/↑	N/↑	N/↓	↓	N/↓	N/↑	N/↑	N/↑	N/↑	N/↑	N/↓
Mitral regurgitation	↑	N/↑	N/↑	↓	↓	N/↑	↑	↑	N/↑	N/↑	↓

Oakes' *Hemodynamic Monitoring: A Bedside Reference Manual*, covers each of the above diseases/disorders in detail, including Definition, Etiology, Pathophysiology, Clinical Manifestations, Hemodynamic Presentation, Diagnostic Studies, and Mgmt.

Major categories are listed above.
All equations are alphabetically listed within each section.

Equation	Comments	Significance
Acid-Base		
Anion Gap	Normal = 12 (± 4) mEq/L	Indicates metabolic acidosis due to an increase of acid (rather than a decrease of base)
1) AG = Na$^+$ – (Cl$^-$ + HCO$_3^-$)		
2) AG = (Na$^+$ + K$^+$) – (Cl$^-$ + HCO$_3^-$)	Normal = 20 (± 4) mEq/L	
	AG = the difference between measured cations (+) and anions (–) (ie., unmeasured ions)	↑ AG = ↑ unmeasured anions (acid): ↑ **acid production**: lactate (hypoxia), ketones (diabetes) ↑ **acid addition**: poisons (methanol, salicylates) ↓ **acid excretion**: renal failure ↓ AG = ↓ unmeasured anions: albumin
	Note: When an Anion Gap Metabolic Acidosis is present, there are various methods used to calculate for additional or mixed metabolic disorders. See Oakes' *ABG Pocket Guide: Interpretation and Management* for more details.	
Base Excess (BE)		Base deficit (BD) = - BE
1) BE = $\dfrac{\Delta PaCO_2 + \Delta pH \times 100}{2}$	$\Delta PaCO_2$ from 40 ΔpH from 7.40 ΔHCO_3 from 24	Accurate only in ranges of: PaCO$_2$: 30-50, pH 7.30-7.50
2) BE ≈ $\Delta PaCO_2$		
3) BE ≈ ΔHCO_3 + 10 ΔpH		

Interpretation and Management

Oakes'
ABG
Pocket Guide

Dana Oakes

Equation	Comments	Significance
Bicarbonate Correction of pH $HCO_3 = (0.2)$body weight $\times$ BD	Corrects to pH 7.40 BD = base deficit	Used to correct for metabolic acidosis.
Henderson-Hasselbach 1) $pH = 6.1 + \log HCO_3 / H_2CO_3$ 2) $pH = 6.1 + \log [HCO_3 / dissolved\ CO_2]$ 3) $pH = 6.1 + \dfrac{total\ CO_2 - 0.03 PaCO_2}{0.03^3 aCO_2}$ 4) $PaCO_2 = \dfrac{total\ CO_2}{0.3 \times [1 - antilog\ (pH - 6.1)]}$	Total $CO_2 = \dfrac{volume\ \%}{2.2}$	Calculation of pH or $PaCO_2$.

Rule of 8's
 	
At: pH $HCO_3 =$
    7.6   8/8 (FaCO2)
    7.5   6/8 (FaCO2)
    7.4   5/8 (PaCO2)
    7.3   4/8 (PaCO2)
    7.2   3/8 (PaCO2)
	Examples: when
	
	pH 7.4, PaCO2 40,
	   $HCO_3 = 5/8\ (40) = 25$
	
	pH 7.3, PaCO2 60,
	   $HCO_3 = 4/8\ (60) = 30$
		Estimate of HCO_3 in relation to pH and $PaCO_2$.

Equation	Comments	Significance
T40 Bicarbonate $T40 = HCO_3 - expected\ \Delta\ HCO_3$	HCO_3 = standard plasma Expected $\Delta HCO_3 = \dfrac{PaCO_2 - 40}{15}$	Used to find a "true" metabolic component in acute hypercapnia.
Winters Formula $PaCO_2$ predicted = $1.54 \times HCO_3 + 8.36\ (\pm 1)$	Measures respiratory compensation for metabolic acidosis.	$PaCO_2$ (actual) > $PaCO_2$ (pred) = mixed acidosis $PaCO_2$ (actual) < $PaCO_2$ (predicted) = respiratory alkalosis
Oxygenation		
A-a Gradient ($PA-aO_2$) ($A-aDO_2$) Alveolar- arterial O_2 tension difference 1) $PA-aO_2 = PAO_2 - PaO_2$	Normal = 10 - 25 mm Hg (air) = 30 - 50mm Hg (100% O_2). Increases with age and FIO_2. PaO_2 is calculated at FIO_2 0.5 breathed x 20 min to get PaO_2 > 150 (100% not used due to ↑ shunt).	Indicates efficiency of gas exchange. Normal values indicate normal shunt. Distinguishes between true shunt and V/Q mismatch. ↑ = shunt, V/Q mismatch, alveolar hypoventilation, or ↓ diffusion. > 350 mm Hg indicative of weaning failure.
2) $PA-aO_2 = 140 - (PaO_2 + PaCO_2)$.	ABG is drawn for $PaCO_2$ and PaO_2.	Less accurate estimate (on 21% only).
3) $PA-aO_2 / 20$	Estimate of shunt (100% O_2)	See shunt equation.

9-4

Equation	Comments	Significance
Alveolar O_2 Tension (Alveolar air equation) (PAO_2)	Normal = 100 mm Hg(air) = 663 mm Hg (100%, sea level)	Partial pressure of O_2 in alveoli. Used to determine alveolar O_2 tension to calculate $PA-aO_2$ gradient, a/A ratio, and % shunt.
1) $PAO_2 = ([PB - PH_2O] \times FIO_2) - PaCO_2 \times (FIO_2 + 1 - FIO_2/RE)$	RE = respiratory exchange ratio (normal = 0.8)	
2) $PAO_2 = ([PB - PH_2O] \times FIO_2) - PaCO_2 (1.25)$	Short form when breathing < 100% O_2	
3) $PAO_2 = PIO_2 - PaCO_2 (1.25)$	Short form when breathing 100% O_2. $PIO_2 = (PB - PH_2O) \times FIO_2$ Estimate only on room air	
4) $PAO_2 = 150 - PaCO_2 (1.25)$	Estimate only	
5) $PAO_2 = (FIO_2 \times 700) - 50$		
Arterial/Alveolar O_2 Tension (a/A Ratio)	Index of gas exchange function or efficiency of the lungs.	More stable than A-a gradient: A-a gradient changes with FIO_2, a/A remains relatively stable with FIO_2 changes. Changes only with $PaCO_2$ or V/Q changes.
PaO_2 / PAO_2	Normal = 0.8 - 0.9 (0.75 elderly) at any FIO_2.	Low a/A (<0.6) = shunt; V/Q mismatch, or diffusion defect; < 0.35 indicative of weaning failure, <0.15 = refractory hypoxemia.
PaO_2 known / PaO_2 calculated = PaO_2 desired / PaO_2 unknown	Useful to predict PaO_2 when changing FIO_2 (See FIO_2 estimation equation)	Can be used to estimate shunt (See shunt equation).

9-5

Equation	Comments	Significance
Arterial-(mixed)Venous O_2 Content Difference $(Ca-\bar{v}O_2)$ $CaO_2 - C\bar{V}O_2 = Ca-\bar{v}O_2$	Difference between arterial and mixed venous O_2 contents. Normal = 4.2 - 5.0 mL/dL (vol%)	Represents O_2 consumption by tissue and estimate of cardiac output. $\uparrow$ = $\downarrow$CO or $\uparrow$ metabolism. $\downarrow$ = $\uparrow$CO or $\downarrow$ metabolism.
Arterial-(mixed)Venous O_2 Tension Difference $(Pa-\bar{v}O_2$ or $a-\bar{v}DO_2)$ $PaO_2 - P\bar{v}O_2 = Pa-\bar{v}O_2$	Normal = 60 mm Hg	Difference between arterial and mixed venous O_2 tensions.
Arterial CO_2 tension (PaCO2) $PaCO_2 = \dfrac{\dot{V}CO_2}{\dot{V}A}$	Normal = 35-45 mm Hg	
FIO2 Estimation 1) Using a/A ratio: $PAO_2 = PaO_2$ desired / a/A ratio	Figured at any FIO_2.	Used to estimate the FIO_2 needed to achieve a desired PaO_2 or the PaO_2 that will be achieved at any given FIO_2.
2)Using alveolar O_2 tension: $FIO_2 = PAO_2 + (PaCO_2 / 0.8) / (PB-H_2O)$	Need $\uparrow FIO_2$ x 20 minutes	$\dfrac{Current\ PaO_2}{Current\ FIO_2} = \dfrac{Desired\ PaO_2}{New\ FIO_2}$
3)Using A-a gradient: $FIO_2 = PA-aO_2 +$ desired PaO_2 /760		$New\ FIO_2 = PaO_2$ desired + $PaCO_2$ desired $/ (PaO_2 / PAO_2) / (PB - H_2O)$
4) Using P/F Ratio: PaO_2 should be: $\dfrac{5\ PaO_2}{1\ FIO_2}$		
5) Estimate: $FIO_2 = PaO_2 / 500$		

9-6

Equation	Comments	Significance
O_2 Consumption (Demand) ($\dot{V}O_2$) $\dot{V}O_2 = CO \times (CaO_2 - C\bar{v}O2) \times 10$ $= CO \times Ca\text{-}\bar{v}O_2 \times 10$	Normal = 200 - 250 mL/min	Volume of O_2 consumed (utilized) by the body tissues per min. Index of metabolic level and CO. $\uparrow\dot{V}O_2 = \uparrow$metabolism or CO; $\downarrow\dot{V}O_2 = \downarrow$metabolism or CO
O_2 Consumption Index ($\dot{V}O_2I$) $\dot{V}O_2I = CI \times Ca\text{-}\bar{v}O_2 \times 10$	$\dot{V}O_2I = \dot{V}O_2/BSA$ $= 110\text{-}165$ mL/min/m²	O_2 consumption per body size.
O_2 Content 1) Arterial $CaO_2 = (Hgb \times 1.36) \times SaO_2 + (PaO_2 \times 0.0031)$	Normal = 15-24 mL/dL (vol%) Both 1.36 and 1.39 are considered correct. Hgb = gm %	Total amount of O_2 in arterial blood (combined plus dissolved).
2) Venous (mixed) $C\bar{v}O_2 = (Hgb \times 1.36) \times S\bar{v}O_2 - (P\bar{v}O_2 \times 0.0031)$ $= \dot{V}O_2/CO$	Normal = 12-15 mL/dL (vol%) $P\bar{v}O_2$ = pressure in mixed venous blood obtained from pulmonary artery.	Total amount of O_2 in mixed venous blood (combined plus dissolved). SaO_2 and $S\bar{v}O_2$ obtained from oximeter or oxyheme dissociation curve.
3) Pulmonary capillary CcO_2	See shunt equation.	

Equation	Comments	Significance
O_2 Delivery (Supply, Transport) ($\dot{D}O_2$) $\dot{D}O_2 = CO \times CaO_2 \times 10$	Normal = 750-1000 mL/min Quantity of O_2 delivered to the body tissues per minute. Requires CO determination.	$\uparrow O_2$ transport = $\uparrow CO$ +/or $\uparrow CaO_2$ $\downarrow O_2$ transport = $\downarrow CO$ +/or $\downarrow CaO_2$ 10 = conversion factor to mL/min
O_2 Delivery Index ($\dot{D}O_2I$) $\dot{D}O_2I = CI \times CaO_2 \times 10$	$\dot{D}O_2I = \dot{D}O_2 / BSA$ = 500-600 mL/min/m²	O_2 delivery per body size.
O_2 Extraction Ratio (O_2 ER) O_2 ER = $\dfrac{O_2 \text{ consumption (demand)}}{O_2 \text{ delivery (supply)}}$ $= \dfrac{\dot{V}O_2 \times 100}{\dot{D}O_2}$ $= \dfrac{Ca\text{-}\bar{v}O_2}{CaO_2}$	Normal = 25 % Amount of O_2 extracted and consumed by the body tissues, relative to the amount delivered. Estimate = $\dfrac{Sa\text{-}\bar{v}O_2}{SaO_2}$	Indicator of O_2 supply/demand balance. $\uparrow$ ratio = $\downarrow FO_2$ +/or $\uparrow O_2$ transport $\downarrow$ ratio = $\uparrow O_2$ +/or $\downarrow O_2$ transport
O_2 Index (OI)	OI = ($\overline{P}aw \times FIO_2 \times 100$) / PaO_2	> 40 = severe respiratory distress with high mortality; 20 - 25 = mortality > 50%
O_2 Reserve O_2 Reserve = $\dot{D}O_2 - \dot{V}O_2$	Normal = 750 mL/min = CO x $Cv̄O_2$ x 10	Venous O_2 supply: O_2 supply minus O_2 demand

9-8

Equation	Comments	Significance
O2 Saturation (mixed venous) (S$\bar{v}$O$_2$) S$\bar{v}$O$_2$ = SaO$_2$ - $\dot{V}$O$_2$/$\dot{D}$O$_2$ = SaO$_2$ - Sa$\bar{v}$O$_2$	Normal = 75 % (60-80 %)	Percent of hemoglobin in mixed venous blood, saturated with O$_2$.
O2 Saturation (SaO$_2$) SaO$_2$ = HbO$_2$/Total Hb x 100	Normal - 95-100% HbO$_2$ = Oxyhemoglobin Content	% of Hemoglobin available that is carrying Oxygen
P/F Ratio (Oxygenation Ratio) PaO$_2$ / FIO$_2$	Normal = 400 – 500 (regardless of FIO$_2$) What PaO$_2$ Should Be: $\frac{5\ PaO_2}{1\ FIO_2}$%	< 300 indicative of ALI < 200 = ARDS
Predicted PaO$_2$ (based on age)	PaO$_2$ = 110 – ½ age	
Respiratory Index (RI) PA-aO$_2$ / PaO$_2$	Normal = < 1.0	1.0- 5.0 = V/Q mismatch > 5.0 = refractory hypoxemia due to physiol. shunt

Equation	Comments	Significance
Respiratory Quotient (Exchange ratio) (RQ, RE, RR) 1) $RQ = \dfrac{\dot{V}CO_2}{\dot{V}O_2}$ 2) $RQ = \dot{V}E \times \dfrac{F\bar{E}\,CO_2 - FICO_2}{FIO_2 - F\bar{E}\,O_2}$ 3) $RQ = \dfrac{F\bar{E}\,CO_2}{FIO_2 - F\bar{E}\,O_2}$	$\dfrac{\text{Volume } CO_2 \text{ produced/min}}{\text{Volume } O_2 \text{ consumed/min}}$ Normal = 200 / 250 = 0.8	RQ = ratio of CO_2 produced to O_2 consumed (internal respiration). RE represents the amount of O_2/CO_2 exchange in the lungs per minute (external respiration). RE = RQ in steady state condition.
Ventilation/Perfusion Index (VQI) $VQI = \dfrac{1 - SaO_2}{1 - S\bar{V}O_2}$	Normal = 0.8	Combines assessment of SaO_2 and $S\bar{V}O_2$ to estimate venous admixture. Correlates well with $\dot{Q}s/\dot{Q}t$.
Ventilation		
Alveolar Ventilation ($\dot{V}A$) 1) $\dot{V}A = \dot{V}E - \dot{V}D$ 2) $\dot{V}A = (V_T - V_{Dphys}) \times f$ 3) $\dot{V}A = (\dot{V}ECO_2 / PaCO_2) \times 863$ 4) Ideal $\dot{V}A = (\dot{V}ECO_2 / PaCO_2$ desired) $\times 863$ 5) $\dot{V}A \times PaCO_2$ known = $\dot{V}A \times$ $PaCO_2$ desired	Normal = 4 - 6 L/min $\dot{V}ECO_2 = \dot{V}E$ measured $\times$ $F\bar{E}\,CO_2$ calculated or measured $F\bar{E}\,CO_2 = P\bar{E}\,CO_2$ measured / $PB - PH_2O$ 863 = correction factor if in milliliters, (0.863 if in liters). Estimated $\dot{V}ECO_2 = 3mL/kg/min$	The volume of inspired air which participates in gas exchange per minute. Used to calculate the ideal alveolar ventilation needed to maintain a desired $PaCO_2$.

Equation	Comments	Significance
Alveolar Volume (V_A)		The volume of each breath that partici-pates in gas exchange.
1) $V_A = \dot{V}_A / f$		
2) $V_A = V_T - V_D$		
3) $V_A = 2 \times IBW$ (lbs)	Estimate	
4) $V_A = 2/3\ V_T$	Estimate (normal)	
Deadspace Ventilation ($\dot{V}_D$)	Normal = $1/3\ \dot{V}_E$	The volume of wasted air (not partici-pating in gas exchange) per minute.
1) $\dot{V}_{Dphys} = V_{Dphys} \times f$		
2) $\dot{V}_{Dphys} = \dot{V}_E - \dot{V}_A$		
3) $\dot{V}_{Dphys} = \left(\dfrac{PaCO_2 - P\bar{E}CO_2}{PaCO_2} \right) \times \dot{V}_E$		
4) $\dot{V}_{Dphys} = \dot{V}_D/V_T \times \dot{V}_E$		
Deadspace Volume (V_D)	Normal = $1/3\ V_T$	The volume of wasted air (not partici-pating in gas exchange) per breath (V > Q).
1) $V_D = V_T - V_A$	V_{Danat} = anatomical V_D (1 mL/lb IBW; 0.5 mL/lb with ET tube or trach)	
2) $V_D = \dot{V}_E - \dot{V}_A / f$	V_{Dalv} = alveolar V_D	$\uparrow V_{Dalv}$ = $\downarrow$ CO, pulmonary vasocon-striction, pulmonary embolus
3) $V_{Dphys} = V_{Danat} + V_{Dalv} + V_{Dmech} + V_{Dcomp}$ = total V_D	V_{Dmech} = mechanical (10mL/inch)	
	V_{Dcomp} = tubing compliance loss	

Equation	Comments	Significance
Deadspace / Tidal Volume Ratio $(V_D/V_T$ Ratio) 1) Bohr Equation: $$\frac{V_{dphys}}{V_T} = \frac{PaCO_2 - P\bar{E}CO_2}{PaCO_2}$$ $$\frac{V_{danat}}{V_T} = \frac{PetCO_2 - P\bar{E}CO_2}{PetCO_2}$$ 2) Estimate: $V_{dphys}/V_T = (\dot{V}_E \text{ actual} / \dot{V}_E \text{ pre-}$ dicted$) \times (PaCO_2 \text{ actual} / 40) \times 0.33$	Normal = 0.33 $\frac{(150\ V_D)}{(450\ V_T)}$ $P\bar{E}CO_2$ = mixed expired Normal = 0.33 (no ABG required) Pet = end tidal This equation is quite accurate. No mixed expired sample required.	Used to measure the portion of V_T not participating in gas exchange (wasted ventilation). $V_D/V_T > 0.5$ is indicative of respiratory failure. Many lung diseases (atelectasis, pneumonia, pulmonary edema, emboli, etc.) can exhibit changes in V_D (i.e., V_{Dalv}) without corresponding changes in $PaCO_2$.
Minute Ventilation ($\dot{V}_E$) (Minute Volume) 1) $\dot{V}_E = V_T \times f$ 2) $\dot{V}_E = \dot{V}_A + \dot{V}_D$ 3) $\dot{V}_E = 1/PaCO_2$ 4) New $\dot{V}_E = \dot{V}_E$ current x $PaCO_2$ current/ $PaCO_2$ desired 5) $PaCO_2$ desired x $\dot{V}_E$ needed = $PaCO_2$ current x $\dot{V}_E$ current 6) Nomogram (See next page)	Normal = 5 - 7 L/min. Changing f is often preferred to changing V_T (due to altering V_D/V_T ratio). $\dot{V}_A$ = effective alveolar ventilation $\dot{V}_D$ = physiological deadspace	The total air in or out of the lungs in one minute. Used to calculate the $\dot{V}_E$ needed to maintain a desired $PaCO_2$. Change rate to change $\dot{V}_E$, changing V_T may alter the V_D/V_T ratio.

Equation	Comments	Significance
Ventilation/Perfusion Ratio ($\dot{V}/\dot{Q}$ Ratio) $$\dot{V}_A/\dot{Q}c = \frac{((C\overline{v}CO_2 - CaCO_2) \times 8.63}{PaCO_2}$$	Normal = $\frac{4L/min}{5L/min}$ = 0.8 Ratio of minute alveolar ventilation to minute capillary blood flow. Represents external respiration.	Ratio changes represent the degree and type of respiratory imbalances. ↓ Ratio (↓$\dot{V}$/$\dot{Q}$) = atelectasis, COPD, pneumonia, pneumothorax, N-M disorders, etc. ↑ Ratio ($\dot{V}$/↑$\dot{Q}$) = shock, pulmonary emboli, cor pulmonale, PPV.

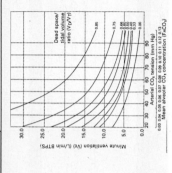

Nomogram to estimate minute ventilation required to maintain a given PaCO2 when VD/VT is known:

To obtain the require minute ventilation to achieve a given
PaCO2, the minute ventilation is plotted against the PaCO2
(measured simultaneously) and the VD/VT ratio is read on the
isopleth that corresponds to the intersection. The isopleth is
then followed to the desired PaCO2 and the corresponding
minute ventilation read off the vertical axis.

For example: A patient with a VE of 5L and a PaCO2 of 60
mmHg has an estimated VD/VT ratio of 0.40. To achieve a
desired PaCO2 of 40 mmHg, follow the 0.40 isopleth up to
correspond to the PaCO2 of 40 on the horizontal axis. Then
read the appropriate minute ventilation of about 8L/min off
the vertical axis.

Equation	Comments	Significance
Ventilator Calculations		
Ventilator Flow $\dot{V} = \dot{V}_E \times RFF$ or $\dot{V} = \dot{V}_E \times 1/TI\%$	RFF = ratio flow factor = I + E Example: I:E ratio = 1:3, RFF = 4	Used to calculate proper flow to deliver a V_T in a given T_I.
Ventilator Rate Needed for Desired $PaCO_2$ New rate = $\dfrac{\text{current rate} \times PaCO_2}{\text{desired } PaCO_2}$	Desired $\dot{V}_E$ = $\dfrac{\text{Current } PaCO_2 \times \text{Current } \dot{V}_E}{\text{desired } PaCO_2}$	This equation holds presuming a steady metabolic rate, stable or no spontaneous breathing, and no change in other ventilator parameters, or Vdmech, or $V_D$mech.
Mechanics		
Airway Occlusion Pressure (P0.1)	Normal = < 2 cm H_2O Change in airway pressure at 0.1 sec after beginning inspiration against an occluded airway. Used to assess ventilatory drive and demand. Indicative of ventilatory demand.	↑ P0.1 = ↑ patient workload +/or drive (possible inadequate ventilator support). ↓ P0.1 = ↓ patient workload +/or drive (possible excessive ventilator support). > 4 - 6 cm H_2O is indicative of weaning failure. (See PImax) Although actual value is negative, it is reported as a positive.

Equation	Comments	Significance
Airway Resistance (R:Raw) 1) $R = \Delta P / \dot{V}$ 2) $Raw = Pmouth - Palv / \dot{V}_I$ 3) $Raw = PIP - Pplat / \dot{V}_I$ 4) $Raw = Cdyn - Cstat$ (see below)	Normal = 0.5 - 2.5 cm H_2O/L/sec @ 0.5 L/sec (30 L/min) ET tube = 4 - 8 cm H_2O/L/sec $\dot{V}_I$ = inspiratory flow in L/sec, square wave flow pattern (use 30 L/min if comparing with norm).	Represents frictional resistance of air-flow (80%) and tissue motion (20%). $Raw \approx 1/r^4$ ↑ airflow resistance = airway collapse, edema, bronchospasm, secretions, ET tube etc. ↑ tissue resistance = pulmonary edema, fibrosis, pneumonia, etc. (see Ch 7). > 5 cm H_2O/L/sec may = wean failure.
Clinical Note: A quick estimate of Raw: = P_{TA} (transairway pressure) = PIP - Pplat ↑P_{TA} = ↑Raw ↓P_{TA} = ↓Raw	↑PIP + ↑Pplat (P_{TA} constant) = ↓Cstat ↑PIP + same Pplat (↑P_{TA}) = ↑Raw ↓PIP + ↓Pplat (P_{TA} constant) = ↑Cstat ↓PIP + same Pplat (↓P_{TA}) = ↓Raw	Pressure support is used primarily to overcome airway resistance of circuit and ET tube. Appropriate PS level can be estimated as PTA (i.e., PIP - Pplat). Note: By convention Raw refers to inspiratory Raw. Expiratory Raw may be determined by PIP - PEEP / $\dot{V}expir$ and is typically > inspiratory Raw.

9-15

Equation	Comments	Significance
Compliance (C) $C = \Delta V / \Delta P$ $C_{LT} = C_L + C_{cw}$ $\quad = \Delta V / Palv - PB$	Normal = 70 - 100 mL/cm H_2O Total compliance is referred to as C_{LT} (lung + thorax) or Crs (respiratory system).	Represents the ease of distention of the lungs and thorax. Includes elastic, functional, and tissue viscous resistance. Ideal = 100mL/ cm H_2O
$C_L = \Delta V / Palv - Ppl$ $C_{cw} = \Delta V / Ppl - PB$	C_L = lung compliance Ccw = chest wall (thorax) compliance	Lungs and chest wall each = 200 mL/ cm H_2O. P_B = barometric pressure; Ppl = pleural pressure Palv = alveolar pressure

9-16

Equation	Comments	Significance
Static Compliance (Cstat)	Normal = 70 - 100 mL/cm H_2O	Represents the combination of lung elasticity and chest wall recoil.
How To Measure $Cstat = V_T - Vtubing / Pplat - PEEP$	Vtubing = volume loss in tubing due to circuit compliance Vtubing = CF (tubing compliance factor) x Pgradient (Pplat - PEEP)	Usually measured while on MV.
Pplat = the pressure needed to maintain lung inflation during zero airflow. It is measured by using either an inspiratory hold or temporarily occluding the exhalation port until pressure stabilizes (approx 1 - 4 sec).	CF must be determined for each patient-ventilator setup (normals range from 1.5 - 5.0 mL/cm H_2O). It is either calculated by newer ventilators or manually by: setting V_T to 200 mL, triggering the ventilator, occluding the patient wye, and observing PIP. CF = $V_T (200) / PIP$	↓ Cstat = ↓ lung elasticity or ↓ chest wall recoil. ↑ Cstat = ↑ lung elasticity or ↑ chest wall recoil. For conditions causing ↑ or ↓ Cstat, see Oakes' *Ventilator Management* book.
$PEEP = PEEPE + PEEPI$	(Pplat can be used in place of PIP). $Vtubing = (V_T (200) / PIP) x (Pplat - PEEP)$	Trend changes in Cstat and Cdyn are more significant in interpreting lung conditions than single measurements.
Clinical Note: In VV, a ↓Cstat results in an ↑PIP and ↑Pplat (V_T constant). In PV, a ↓Cstat results in a ↓V_T (PIP and Pplat constant).		A Cstat ≤ 25- 33 mL/cm H_2O is indicative of weaning failure. Cstat can also be used to determine optimal PEEP.

Equation	Comments	Significance
Dynamic Compliance (Cdyn)	Normal = 40 - 70 mL/cm H_2O	Represents the combination of static lung compliance (Cstat) and airway resistance (Raw).
How To Measure	Vtubing = CF x (PIP - PEEP) (See Cstat above to determine CF)	For conditions causing $\uparrow$ or $\downarrow$ Cdyn, see Cstat (above)
Cdyn = V_T - Vtubing / PIP - PEEP	PEEP = $PEEP_E$ + $PEEP_I$	Trend changes in Cstat and Cdyn are more significant in interpreting lung conditions than single measurements.
Usually measured while on MV.		

Clinical Notes:

$\uparrow$Cdyn (same Cstat) = $\downarrow$Raw
$\downarrow$Cdyn (same Cstat) = $\uparrow$Raw

In VV, a $\downarrow$ Cdyn results in an $\uparrow$PIP (V_T constant).
In VV, a $\downarrow$PIP (V_T constant) = improved Cstat or Raw or a leak.

$\uparrow$Cdyn (with same$\uparrow$ in Cstat) = $\uparrow$Cstat
$\downarrow$Cdyn (with same $\downarrow$ in Cstat) = $\downarrow$Cstat

In PV, a $\downarrow$Cdyn results in a $\downarrow V_T$ (PIP constant).
In PV, an $\uparrow V_T$ (PIP constant) = improved Cstat or Raw.

$\uparrow$Cdyn (with partial $\uparrow$ in Cstat) = $\downarrow$Raw and $\uparrow$Cstat
$\downarrow$Cdyn (with partial $\downarrow$ in Cstat) = $\uparrow$Raw and $\downarrow$Cstat

9-18

Equation	Comments	Significance
Equation of Motion $Pawo = V/C + (Raw \times \dot{V})$	Elastic components of respiratory system: $P = V/C$ $V = P \times C$ $C = V/P$ Resistive components of respiratory system: $P = Raw \times \dot{V}$ $\dot{V} = P/Raw$ $Raw = P/\dot{V}$	At any moment the airway opening pressure (Pawo) must exactly balance the opposing lung and chest wall expansion forces. P, $\dot{V}$, I, + V can be controlled by the clinician. In VV: Set $\dot{V}$: P varies with Raw Set V: P varies with C In PV: Set P: $\dot{V}$ varies with Raw Set P: V varies with C
Maximal Inspiratory Pressure (PImax) (MIP, NIP) Two methods: Marini #1- total occlusion @ end-exhalation Marini #2- total occlusion @ below FRC	The maximal inspiratory effort (pressure) generated against an occluded airway (approx 20 sec). Normal < 20 cm H_2O (i.e., < - 20 cm H_2O) Although actual value is negative, it is reported as a positive.	Indicative of the capability of the inspiratory muscles. (See P0.1 above) P0.1 / PImax = demand / capability = predictive weaning index ≤ 0.9 indicative of weaning failure Prior to start of test patient should be actively breathing (remove vent support). Remove PEEPe and PEEPi. Respiratory muscles should not be fatigued.

Equation	Comments	Significance
Mean Airway Pressure ($\overline{P}aw$) $\overline{P}aw = \dfrac{(T_I \times PIP) + (T_E \times PEEP)}{T_{tot}}$ $\overline{P}aw = (PIP - PEEP) \times T_I/T_{tot} + PEEP$	Average airway pressure during several breathing cycles.	$\overline{P}aw = ([P_{TA} + \frac{1}{2} PA] - PEEP) \times T_I/T_{tot} + PEEP$ Note: Should always be less than CVP (1 cm H_2O = 0.735 mmHg)
Rapid - Shallow Breathing Index (RSBI) $RSBI = f/V_T$ or $f^2/\dot{V}_E$	Measure f and V_T (in liters) while off the ventilator. Normal = < 100	Has proven to be one of the best predictive indices for weaning. > 105 is indicative of weaning failure
Time Constant (TC) $TC = Raw \times Cstat$ $TC = \Delta P/\dot{V} \times \Delta V/\Delta P$ Note: TC generally refers to inspiratory TC. Expiratory TC may be much longer than inspiratory TC in COPD.	1TC = 63% 2TC = 87% 3TC = 95% 4TC = 98% 5TC = 99% % = % of V_T entering lungs within each TC period. Normal TC = 0.2 sec Normal T_I = 3 - 4 TC = 3 or 4 x 0.2 sec = 0.6 – 0.8 sec	TC (inspir) indicates alveolar filling time. ↑TC (> 0.2 sec) is usually indicative of ↑Raw (but may be ↑C_{LT}). ↓TC (< 0.2 sec) is usually indicative of ↓C_{LT} (but may be ↓Raw). TC(expir) indicates alveolar emptying time. < 3 TCexpir will generally result in air-trapping. TCexpir may be approximated with a F-V loop.

Equation	Comments	Significance
Vital Capacity (VC)	Normal is 60-80 mL/kg	< 60 mL/kg indicates general restr. process > 10 mL/kg is needed for effective deep breathing and cough. < 10 mL/kg = impending respiratory failure
Work of Breathing (WCB) $W = \int P \times V$ WOB / min (W) = WOB $\times$ f WOB / liter = W / $\dot{V}_E$ WOB total = WOB patient + WOB vent	The energy (pressure gradient) required to take a breath. Normal = 0.6 - 1.0 j (1j = 0.1 kg.m) W / $\dot{V}_E$ closely reflects abnormal pulmonary mechanics.	Intrinsic WOB = energy required to overcome patient's elastic and resistive forces. Extrinsic WOB = energy required to overcome added extrinsic systems
Weaning Equations		
CROP CROP = Cdyn x (PaO$_2$/PAO$_2$) x PImax / rate	C = compliance R = rate O = oxygenation P = pressure	< 13 mL/breath/min indicative of weaning failure.
Simplified Weaning Index SWI = f (mech) x (PIP - PEEP / PImax) x (PaCO$_2$ / 40)	Normal = < 9 min	Simplified version of weaning index (WI). Less accurate than WI, but quick and easy. > 11 min indicative of weaning failure
P0.1 / PImax and RSBI (f /V$_T$): See above		

9-21

Equation	Comments	Significance
Perfusion/Hemodynamic Monitoring		
Cardiac Index (CI) $CI = CO/BSA$	Cardiac output per body size. Normal = 2.5 - 4.4 L/min/m^2 BSA (See Pg 9-28)	More precise measure of pump efficiency than CO. CI 1.8 - 2.5 = moderate cardiac disease CI < 1.8 = severe cardiac disease
Cardiac Output (CO or $\dot{Q}_T$) $CO = SV \times HR$	Normal = 4-8 L/min (at rest) See Fick equation below & Oakes' ***Hemodynamic Monitoring: A Bedside Reference Manual*** for more information.	Amount of blood ejected from heart per minute. Indicator of pump efficiency and a determinant of tissue perfusion.
Coronary Artery Perfusion Pressure (CPP or CAPP) $CPP = MAP - PAWP$ $= BPdia - PAWP$	Normal = 60-80 mm Hg	Driving pressure of coronary blood flow.
Fick Equation $\dot{V}O_2 = CO \times Ca\text{-}\bar{v}O_2$	See Oakes' ***Hemodynamic Monitoring: A Bedside Reference Manual*** for more info.	Method of measuring cardiac output. Fick estimate: $CO = 125 \times BSA / Ca\text{-}\bar{v}O_2$

Equation	Comments	Significance
Left Ventricular Stroke Work (LVSW) LVSW = $(\overline{BP} - PAWP)$ x SV x 0.0136	Normal = 60-80 gm/m/beat	Measure of pumping function of left ventricle (LV contractility).
Left Ventricular Stroke Work Index (LVSWI) LVSWI = $(\overline{BP} - PAWP)$ x SVI x 0.0136	Normal = 40-75 gm/m/beat/m^2	Measure of pumping function of left ventricle (LV contractility) / body size.
Mean Arterial Blood Pressure $(\overline{BP},\ MAP)$ $\overline{BP}$ = 1/3 PP + BPdia = $\dfrac{BP_{sys} + 2BP_{dia}}{3}$	Normal = 93 mm Hg (70-105)	Average driving force of systemic circulation. Determined by cardiac output and total peripheral resistance.
Mean Pulmonary Artery Pressure $(\overline{PAP},\ PAMP)$ $\overline{PAP}$ = 1/3 pulmPP + PADP	Normal = 10 - 15 mm Hg = $\dfrac{PASP + 2PADP}{3}$	Average driving force of blood from the right heart to left heart.
Pulmonary Vascular Resistance (PVR) PVR = $\dfrac{PAMP - PAWP}{CO}$ x 80	Normal = 20-250 dynes•sec•cm^{-5} = 0.25-2.5 units (mm Hg/L/min) E.g. $\dfrac{14\ mm\ Hg - 5\ mm\ Hg}{5\ L/min}$ = 1.8 units mm Hg/L/min x 80 = dynes•sec•cm^{-5}	Resistance to RV ejection of blood into pulmonary vasculature. Indicator of RV afterload.

9-23

Equation	Comments	Significance
Pulmonary Vascular Resistance Index (PVRI) $PVRI = \dfrac{PAMP - PAWP}{CI} \times 80$	Normal = 35-350 dynes•sec•cm^{-5}/ m^2	PVR related to body size.
Pulse Pressure (PP) $PP = BP_{sys} - BP_{dia}$	Normal = 40 mm Hg (20-80)	Difference between BP systolic and BP diastolic.
Rate Pressure Product (RPP) $RPP = BP_{sys} \times HR$	Normal = < 12,000 mm Hg/min	Indirect determinant of M$\dot{V}O_2$.
Right Ventricular Stroke Work (RVSW) = $(PAMP - CVP) \times SV \times 0.0136$	Normal = 10-15 gm/m/beat	Measure of pumping function of right ventricle (RV contractility).
Right Ventricular Stroke Work Index (RVSW) = $(PAMP - CVP) \times SVI \times 0.0136$ = RVSW / BSA	Normal = 4-12 gm/m/beat/m^2	Measure of pumping function of right ventricle (RV contractility) / body size.

Equation	Comments	Significance

Shunt Equation ($\dot{Q}_s / \dot{Q}_T$)
 	
1) Classical
$$\dot{Q}_s / \dot{Q}_T = \frac{Cc_{O_2} - Ca_{O_2}}{Cc - \overline{v}_{O_2}}$$
	Normal = 2-5%
	Cc_{O_2} = pulmonary capillary blood O_2 content ("ideal") at 100% saturated with alveolar O_2. Cannot be sampled.
	Cc_{O_2} = (Hgb x 1.34) Sa_{O_2} + (Pa_{O_2} x 0.003)
		Indicates ratio of shunted blood (Q_s) (blood not participating in gas exchange) to total cardiac output (Q_T).
		$Q_s = Q_T - Q_c$
		$Q_s = Q_{sphys} = Q_{sanat} + Q_{scap}$
		Indicator or efficiency of pulm system:
		  < 10% = normal lungs
		  10-20% = minimal effect
		  20-30% = significant pulm disease
		  > 30% = life-threatening

2) Clinical $$\dot{Q}_s / \dot{Q}_T = \frac{PA\text{-}a_{O_2} \times 0.003}{Ca\text{-}\overline{v}_{O_2} + PA\text{-}a_{O_2} \times 0.003}$$	Less accurate/easier. Perform breathing ↑ FIO_2 (50% preferred over 100% due to ↑shunting from alveolar collapse) x 20 minutes.	Clinical equation assumes Hgb 100% saturated ($Pa_{O_2} > 150$). If $Pa_{O_2} < 150$, then must use classical shunt equation. Ca-$\overline{v}_{O_2}$ can be assumed if a mixed venous sample cannot be obtained: 4.5 - 5% in patients with good CO and perfusion. 3.5% in critically ill patients.
3) Estimate $$\dot{Q}_s / \dot{Q}_T = \frac{PA\text{-}a_{O_2} \times 0.003}{3.5 + PA\text{-}a_{O_2} \times 0.003}$$	5%/100 mm Hg (2%/50 mm Hg) Most accurate when breathing 100% O_2. Plus normal 2-5%. Estimate good until $Pa_{O_2} < 100$ mm Hg	Estimate: $Pa_{O_2}/FIO_2 > 300$ = < 15% shunt 200 - 300 = 15 - 20%; < 200 = > 20% shunt
4) Estimates $$\dot{Q}_s / \dot{Q}_T = \frac{PA\text{-}a_{O_2}}{20}$$ $\dot{Q}_s / \dot{Q}_T$ = 5% per ≥very 100 mm Hg be ow expected	5%/100 mm Hg (2%/50 mm Hg) Most accurate when breathing 100% O_2. Plus normal 2-5%. Estimate good until $Pa_{O_2} < 100$ mm Hg	Estimate: $Pa_{O_2}/FIO_2 > 300$ = < 15% shunt 200 - 300 = 15 - 20%; < 200 = > 20% shunt

9-25

Equation	Comments	Significance
Stroke Volume (SV) $SV = CO/HR \times 1000$	Normal = 60-120 mL/beat	Amount of blood ejected by either ventricle per contraction.
Stroke Volume Index (SVI) $SVI = CO/HR \times 1000 / BSA$	Normal = 35-75 mL/beat/m^2	Relates SV to body size.
Systemic Vascular Resistance (SVR) $SVR = \dfrac{\overline{BP} - CVP \times 80}{CO}$	Normal = 800-1600 dynes•sec•cm^{-5} = 10-20 units (mm Hg/L/min) E.g. $\dfrac{93 \text{ mm Hg} - 3 \text{ mm Hg} = 18 \text{ units}}{5 \text{ L/min}}$	Resistance to LV ejection of blood into systemic circulation. Indicator of LV afterload. mm Hg/L/min x 80 = dynes•sec•cm^{-5}
Systemic Vascular Resistance Index (SVRI) $SVRI = \dfrac{\overline{BP} - CVP \times 80}{CI}$	Normal = 1400-2600 dynes•sec•cm^{-5}/ m^2	SVR per body size.
Patient Calculations		
Body Surface Area (BSA) $BSA (m^2) = (4 \times Kg) + 7 / Kg + 90$ $BSA (m^2) = (Ht (cm)^{0.725}) \times (Wt (kg)^{0.425}) \times .007184$	BSA (m^2) = $(4 \times Kg) + 7 / Kg + 90$	Used to determine cardiac index and other hemodynamic parameters. Relates parameters to body size. Kg = 2.2 lbs

Equation		Comments	Significance
Ideal Body Weight (IBW)	**SHORTCUT:**	Male: 106 lbs for 5 ft tall. Add 6 lbs/in above 5 ft.	Female: 100 lbs for 5 ft tall. Add 5 lbs/in above 5 ft.
Kg = 2.2 lbs	**ARDS NET:**	Wt [kg] = 50.0 + 0.91 (Ht [cm] - 152.4)	Wt [kg] = 45.5 + 0.91 (Ht [cm] - 152.4)
Pulmonary Function (Bedside)			
% Predicted		$\dfrac{Actual}{Predicted}$ x 100	
% Change		$\dfrac{Post\ Value - Pre\ value}{Pre\ Value}$ x 100	
Miscellaneous			
ATPS to BTPS Vol BTPS = Vol ATPS x factor		See Appendix	Correction of lung volumes measured at room temp to body temp.
Fick's Law of Diffusion Diffusion = $\dfrac{Area\ x\ diffusion\ coefficient\ x\ \Delta P}{Thickness}$			Gas diffusion rate across the lung membrane.

Equation	Comments	Significance
Gas Laws Dalton's Law: $\text{Total P} = P_1 + P_2 + P_3$, etc. Boyle's Law: $P_1 \times V_1 = P_2 \times V_2$ Charles' Law: $V_1/T_1 = V_2/T_2$ Gay-Lussac's Law: $P_1/T_1 = P_2/T_2$ Combined Gas Law: $P_1 \times V_1 / T_1 = P_2 \times V_2 / T_2$	P and V are inversely related (T constant) V and T are directly related (P constant) P and T are directly related (V constant)	
Graham's Law of Diffusion Coefficient	Diffusion coefficient = $\dfrac{\text{solubility coefficient}}{\sqrt{gmw}}$	Rate of gas diffusion is inversely proportional to the square root of its gram molecular weight.
Helium/Oxygen (He/O2) Flow Conversion and Duration	80% He / 20% O2: actual flow = flow × 1.8 70% He / 30% O2 = flow × 1.6 60% He / 40% O2 = flow × 1.4 Duration Factor (see next page, O2)	Conversion is used when an O2 flow meter is used to measure flow. Used in patients with obstructive disorders.
Law of LaPlace	$P = 2ST / r$	P = pressure (dynes/cm²); r = radius (cm) ST = surface tension (dynes/cm)

Equation	Comments	Significance

Oxygen Blending Ratios

$$100 \xrightarrow[\text{air units} \quad \text{O}_2 \text{ units}]{\text{FIO}_2: \text{ desired}} 21$$

Comments:
Select desired FIO$_2$.
Subtract 100 - FIO$_2$ = air units
Subtract FIO$_2$ - 20 = O$_2$ units

Significance:
To find air/O$_2$ ratio for desired FIO$_2$.
Air units/O$_2$ units = air/O$_2$ ratio

E.g: 40% O$_2$ desired

$$\frac{100 - 40 = 60}{40 - 20 = 20} = \frac{60}{20} = \frac{3}{1}$$

Oxygen Duration Times

Duration of a Cylinder

$$\text{Time (min)} = \frac{\text{Pcyl} \times \text{CF}}{\text{Flow (L/min)}}$$

Comments:
Pcyl = total pressure in cylinder (psi) – 500 psi (reserve)

CF = conversion factor (L/psi)
$$= \frac{(\text{ft}^3 \text{ of cyl}) \times 28.3 \text{ L/ft}^3}{\text{max Pcyl}}$$

Heliox H Cylinder Duration Factor:
2.50

O2/CO2 H Cylinder Duration Factor:
3.84

Significance:
Used to calculate how long a cylinder of O$_2$ gas will last. 500 psi equals reserve.

Size (Aluminum)	PSIG	factor
A	2216	0.035
B	2216	0.068
D	2015	0.16
E	2015	0.28
E (Heliox)		0.23
E (Carbogen)		0.35
G		2.41
H/K	2265	3.14
H (Heliox)		2.50
H (Carbogen)		3.84
M	2216	1.65

Equation	Comments	Significance
Duration of a Liquid System	Liquid weight is known: Duration time (min) = $$\frac{344 \text{ L/lb} \times \text{liquid weight (lb)}}{O_2 \text{ flow (L/min)}}$$ 1 L liquid = 860 L gas Liquid Wt = Total Wt - Cylinder Wt	Gauge fraction is known: Duration time (min) = $$\frac{\text{Liquid capacity (L)} \times 860 \times \text{gauge fraction}}{O_2 \text{ flow (L/min)}}$$ Does not account for evaporative loss.
Oxygen Entrainment Ratios $$TF = \frac{O_2 \text{ flow} \times 0.79}{FIO_2 - 0.21}$$ $$FIO_2 = \frac{0.79}{TF / O_2 \text{ Flow}} + 0.21$$	TF = total flow in liters (O_2 + air) Mixture = O_2 + air $(FIO_2)(\text{Flow}) = (1.0)(O_2 \text{ Flow}) + (0.21)(\text{air Flow})$	Determines total flows, entrained flows, or O_2 percent when air and O_2 are entrained together. See O_2 blending ratio above.
Poiseuille's Law $$\dot{V} = \frac{\Delta P \, r \, 4\pi}{\mu L 8} = \frac{\Delta P \, r \, 4}{}$$	$\dot{V}$ = flow, πP = driving pressure 8 = constant, r = radius of airway π = pi	μ = viscosity of gas L = length of airway

9-30

Equation	Comments	Significance
Reynold's Number $Rn = \dfrac{v \times D \times d}{\mu}$	Rn = Reynold's # v = velocity of fluid D = density of fluid	d = diameter of tube μ = viscosity of fluid $Rn < 2000$ = laminar flow $Rn > 2000$ = turbulent
Temperature Conversion	$F^\circ = (C^\circ \times 9/5) + 32^\circ$ $C^\circ = (F^\circ - 32) \times 5/9$	See Appendix $K^\circ = C^\circ + 273$
Tobacco Use (Pack Years)	# Packs Smoked per Day x # Yrs Smkd	- There are usually 20 cigarettes/pk

10 RESPIRATORY PROCEDURES

CONTENTS

PROCEDURES

▶ Indicates AARC Clinical Practice Guideline

Continued on Next Page

▶ Indicates AARC Clinical Practice Guideline

Continued on Next Page

PROCEDURES

AEROSOL THERAPY

Types of Aerosol Therapy	**Bland Aerosol Delivery** (see AARC CPG, Next Page)
	Medicated Aerosol Delivery (See Also Chapter 12)

Hazards of Aerosol Therapy

- Adverse reaction to medication
- Airway obstruction (swollen mucus)
- Airway thermal injury
- Caregiver exposure to airborne contagion
- Bronchospasm
- Drug reconcentration
- Infection
- Overhydration (hypernatremia)
- Overmobilization of secretions
- Systemic effects

Bland Aerosol Administration[1,2]
(AARC CPG)

Indications

A bypassed upper airway (heated bland aerosol, MMAD 2-10 μ) [3]

Mobilization of secretions

Sputum induction (hypo or hypertonic saline, MMAD 1-5μ)

Upper airway edema – (cool bland aerosol, MMAD ≥ 5μ):
Laryngotracheobronchitis
Subglottic edema
Post extubation edema
Post-op management

Assessment of Need

One or more of stridor, croupy cough, hoarseness following extubation, Hx of upper airway irritation with ↑ WOB, LTB or croup, bypassed airway, or patient discomfort.

Hazards/Complications

Bronchoconstriction or wheezing: artificial airway or hyperton. sputum induction in COPD, asthma, CF, other)

Caregiver exposure to airborne contagion

Edema of airway wall or assoc. with ↓C + ↑Raw

Infection

Overhydration

Patient discomfort

Contraindications

Bronchoconstriction

History of airway hyper-responsiveness

Monitoring

Patient:

Respiratory – rate, pattern, mechanics, accessory muscle use, BS.

CV – rate, rhythm, BP

Response – pain, dyspnea, discomfort, restlessness.

Sputum – quantity, color, consistency, odor

Skin color

Pulse oximetry (if hypoxemia suspected)

Equipment – Spirometry if concern of adverse reaction.

Frequency

Post extubation – 4-8 hrs

Subglottic edema – until edema subsides

Bypassed upper airway – as long as bypassed

Sputum induction – prn

Clinical Goals

Water, hypo or isotonic saline:
↓ dyspnea, stridor, or WOB
Improved ABGs, O₂ Sat, or VS

Hypertonic saline: sputum sample

---

1) Bland aerosol therapy is the administration of sterile water, hypotonic, isotonic or hypertonic saline with or without oxygen.

2) Adapted from the AARC Clinical Practice Guideline: Bland Aerosol Administration, 2003 Revision and Update, *Respiratory Care*, Vol. 48, #5, 2003.

3) Not as effective as heated water nebulizers or HME.

Aerosol Delivery Devices

Type	Use	Comments
Small Volume Nebulizer (SVN) *Also called handheld, mini-neb, mainstream, sidestream, slipstream, or in-line*	Used to deliver intermittent aerosolized medications Short-term use only Usually 2-5 mL of solution Optimal gas flow rates 6-8 L/min Average particle size 1-5 μm dia	Can be used with a mouthpiece, face mask, trach-collar, T-piece, or ventilator circuit, with normal breathing pattern and with all patients Need electrical, battery, or gas source to power Requires drug preparation Units can be either pneumatic or ultrasonic Use air, not oxygen, for patients on a hypoxic drive. Patient should take periodic deep breaths
Large Volume Nebulizer (LVN) (jet)	Used for continuous oxygen +/or aerosol therapy (heated or cool). Variable particle size 1-2 mL/min output	Can be used with a face mask, trach-collar, or T-piece. Condensation collects in tubing Correct solution level must be maintained ↑risk of nosocomial infection See air entrainment neb for air/O2 ratios, total $\dot{V}$ Used primarily for patients with tracheostomies.
Ultrasonic (USN)	Used to mobilize thick secretions in the lower airways 90% of particles are 1-5 μm dia Usually only intermittent, but may be continuous therapy. 1- 6 mL/min output	Drug preparation required Heat generated by USN may affect bronchodilators May precipitate bronchospasm, overmobilization of secretions, or overhydration. Not all drugs (e.g., Budesonide and Dornase) are compatible with ultrasonic nebulizers. Provides 100% humidity (continuous)

10-6

Type	Use	Comments
Metered Dose Inhaler (MDI)	Intermittent delivery of aerosolized medications. Particle size 3-6 µm	First method of choice. Small, easily cleaned Efficacy is design and technique dependent Inexpensive, convenient, portable, and no drug prep required Inspiratory flow rates should be ≤ 30 LPM May be used in-line with ventilators Patient self-administered, hence may not be appropriate for pediatric or geriatric patients. Requires hand-breath coordination, synchronization with inspiration, and a 4-10 sec. breath hold. Spacer or holding chamber is recommended, esp. with children.
Dry Powder Inhaler (DPI)	Intermittent delivery of a powdered medication. Particle size 1-2 µm	Breath actuated and patient self-administered Breath holding not required High humidity may affect some drugs. Many drugs unavailable in DPI form Not recommended for patients < 6 yrs or with acute bronchospasm Some units require high flow rates (> 40 Lpm), hence may not be appropriate for pediatric or geriatric patients.
Small Particle Aerosol Generator (SPAG)	Delivery of aerosolized ribavirin.	Specific for ribavirin Caregiver precautions required

Device Selection

- ACCP and ACAAI evidence-based guidelines indicate that all aerosolized delivery systems are equally effective when used properly (Chest Jan, 2005).
- Selection should be based on drug availability, patient's abilities (cognitive, physical, learning, etc), patient preference, convenience, and cost.
- Selection of a specific device should be based on its ability to produce particles with a mass median aerodynamic diameter (MMAD) of 1-3 microns.

Overview

- CDC recommends that nebulizers be filled with sterile fluids (not tap or distilled H_2O), and be changed or replaced q 24 hrs.
- Cost, convenience, and the ease-of-use can affect compliance.
- Patient assessment before, during, and after therapy should include BS, breathing pattern, heart rate, overall appearance, and peak flow for patients with reactive airways.
- The efficacy of inhaled drugs can be affected by the device, the inhalation technique, severity of disease, and patient age.
- Unit dose (vs. multidose bottled) medications should be used.

Nebulizers

- Heated nebs require sterile solution and sterile immersion heaters, if used. Heaters must be monitored for proper funct.
- Nebulizers should be cleaned and changed periodically according to manufacturer recommendations.
- SVNs should be shaken, rinsed with either sterile or distilled water (not tap water), and left to air dry after each use. Drying may be enhanced by gas flow through the device after rinsing.

Newer types of nebulizers that are being studied or recently introduced into clinical practice include:

- Improvements in jet-nebulization (breath-actuated nebulizers)
- Vibrating mesh (porous membrane vibrating at ultrasonic frequencies)
- Pressurized liquids through a nozzle

These newer types of devices use less medication, are more efficient in aerosol delivery, and have little or no deadspace volume.

Metered Dose Inhalers (MDI's)

- **Counting**: Patients should be instructed to keep a tally of actuations used (including "wasted ones"), NOT by placing in a bowl of water.
- MDIs with a holding chamber or spacer reduces the need for patient coordination and improves particle deposition.
- MDI mouthpieces should be washed with mild soap and water every few days.
- Patient instruction and proper usage determines optimal delivery, and periodic assessment of proper technique is important.

MDI Technique
(see Pharmacology Chapter for device-specific information)

	Without Accessory Device		With Accessory Device
1.	Assemble MDI, warm to body temperature		
2.	Inspect mouthpiece for foreign matter		
3.	Shake canister vigorously 3-4 shakes		
4.	If > 24 hrs since last use, deliver one puff into the air (2-4 puffs if first use)	4a.	Attach accessory device (spacer/holding chamber)
5.	Hold MDI upright and sit upright	b.	Place mouthpiece or mask into accessory device
6.	Place mouthpiece 4 cm from open mouth (or between sealed lips for breath actuated device)	c.	Place valve stem into canister holding orifice on accessory device
7.	Exhale normally		
8.	Inspire slowly while depressing MDI canister at same time (inspiratory flow rate < 30 L/m or > 30 for breath actuated).	8a.	If chamber is equipped with a reed device, prevent making a sound during inspiration.
9.	Continue inspiration until TLC		
10	Hold breath 4-10 sec		It is recommended that patients utilize a Spacer, but both techniques be taught for times when a pt doesn't have a spacer, or is noncompliant with spacer use.
11.	Wait 15-30 sec between puffs depending on medication (2 – 10 min for bronchodilators to enhance the effectiveness).		
12.	Repeat as prescribed.		
13.	Rinse mouth after use (esp. with corticosteroid use).		

Dry Powder Inhalers (DPI's)

Patient Instruction:
- Instruct patient to follow Doctor's orders precisely (# and freq. of treatments, medication dosage).
- Patient should be in sitting or high Fowler's position during therapy.
- Patients should be instructed in detecting any possible adverse reactions (see Pharmacology Chapter).
- Many times, Dry Powders do not have taste or texture - pt should be instructed that with proper technique, medication has been delivered despite no sensation to verify that.
- Patients should be instructed to cough, expectorate, or suction as needed.

Clinicians Should:
- Be familiar with the device and practiced with a placebo prior to instructing patients.
- Demonstrate assembly and correct use of device to patients.
- Per device specifications, clinician should verify pt's ability to use device - include inspiratory ability, as well as ability to coordinate/actuate.
- Provide written instructions on how to use the device and a written plan for use.
- Observe patient practice use of the device.

DPI Technique:

1. Assemble DPI and inspect mouthpiece for foreign matter
2. Load the medication (see device instructions)
3. Exhale normally (away from device)
4. Instruct pt to place mouthpiece in mouth, with lips sealed tightly, and inspire per manufacturer recommendations (some devices require short, quick inspiration while others require gradual inspiration)
5. Generally, inspiratory flow rate should be > 60 LPM
6. Hold breath 4-10 seconds
7. Repeat as prescribed
8. Rinse mouth after use (esp. with corticosteroid use).

Effective aerosol therapy requires the correct matching of appropriate device with the patient's ability to use it properly.

Selected Resources:

Respiratory Therapists	• **A Guide to Aerosol Delivery Devices for Respiratory Therapists**; Ari, Hess, Meyers & Rau; AARC (2nd Edition)
	• **AARC Clinical Practice Guidelines:** (see summaries pgs 10-5, 10-12)
	  • Bland Aerosol Administration 2003 Revision and Update
	  • Selection of a Device for Delivery of Aerosol to the Lung Parenchyma
	• **American College of Chest Physicians** (ACCP)
	  • Device Selection and Outcomes of Aerosol Therapy: Evidence-Based Guidelines, 2005

Health Care Professionals	• **Guide to Aerosol Delivery Devices: For Physicians, Nurses, Pharmacists, and Other Health Care Professionals**; Elliot and Dunne; AARC (1st Edition, 2011)
Patients	• **A Patient's Guide to Aerosol Drug Delivery**; Galvin, Dunne and Kallstrom; AARC (1st Edition, 2010)

Recommended particle sizes:

1-5 μ	sputum induction
2-5 μ	pharmacologically active aerosols
2-10 μ	bypassed upper airway
> 5 μ	upper airway administration

MMAD = mass medium aerodynamic diameter (μ)

It is important to again remember that MMAD can be affected by improper patient technique, resulting in inertial impaction, and ultimately less therapeutic deposition.

Selection of a Device for Delivery of Aerosol to the Lung Parenchyma[1] (AARC CPG)

Indication
The need to deliver a topical medication (in aerosol form) that has its site of action in the lung parenchyma or is intended for systemic absorption.

Contraindications
None, medication contraindications may exist.

Hazards/Complications
Malfunction of device, improper technique, medication complications, nebulizer design and characteristics of the medication may affect ventilator function and medication deposition, aerosols may cause bronchospasm or irritation of the airway, exposure to medications and patient-generated droplet nuclei may be hazardous to clinicians

Limitations
Efficacy of device is design and technique dependent, a relatively small fraction of nebulizer output deposits in the lung parenchyma (may be affected by MV, artificial airways, reduced airway caliber (eg, infants and pediatrics)

severity of obstruction, hydrophilic formulations, failure of patient to comply with procedure.

Assessment of Need
Availability of drug, formulation and equipment; superiority of any one method not established; cost, convenience, effectiveness, and patient tolerance of procedure should be considered; consider augmenting with MV when spontaneous ventilation is inadequate.

Assessment of Outcome/ Monitoring
Proper technique, compliance, response of patient, a positive clinical outcome.

Infection Control
Universal precautions, nebulizers should not be used between patients without disinfection, nebulizers should be changed or sterilized at conclusion of dose admin or every 24 hours; at 24-hour intervals with continuous admin; when visibly soiled.

CONTINUED ON NEXT PAGE

Selection of an Aerosol Delivery Device[1]	
continued	
Infection Control, cont. Nebulizers should not be rinsed with tap water between tx, but may be rinsed with sterile water. CDC recommends sterile water rinsing and air drying. All medications should be handled aseptically.	

1) Adapted from AARC Clinical Practice Guideline: Selection of a Device for Delivery of Aerosol to the Lung Parenchyma, *Respiratory Care*, Volume 41, 1996.

For AARC CPG on Assessing Response to Bronchodilator Therapy, see Chapter 12.

Additional Resources

See Oakes' **RespiratoryUpdate.com** for further information
and explanations of Aerosol Therapy, including direct links to:

Books
- A Guide to Aerosol Delivery Devices for Respiratory Therapists
- Guide to Aerosol Delivery Devices: For Physicians, Nurses, Pharmacists, and other Health Care Professionals
- A Patient's Guide to Aerosol Drug Delivery

Evidence-Based Guidelines
American College of Chest Physicians (ACCP)
- Device Selection and Outcomes of Aerosol Therapy: Evidence-Based Guidelines

American Association of Respiratory Care (AARC)
- Assessing Response to Bronchodilator Therapy at Point of Care
- Bland Aerosol Administration 2003 Revision & Update
- Selection of a Device for Delivery of Aerosol to the Lung Parenchyma
- Selection of Device, Administration of Bronchodilator, and Evaluation of Response to Therapy in Mechanically Ventilated Patients

Journal Articles and Teachings to include:
- An AARC Journal Conference on MDIs and DPIs
- Websites devoted to Aerosol Medicine
- Patient instructions and technique videos for inhaled devices
- And more

V **RESPIRATORY UPDATE**

THE Virtual Critical Care Library

Artificial Airways

Types and Indications

Type	Notes	Ventilation	Obstruction	Protection	Secretion
		Indications			
Oro-pharyngeal	Use only in unconscious patients with no cough or gag	X	X		X
Naso-pharyngeal	Useful in pts with (or at risk for developing) airway obstruction (particularly clenched jaw) May be better tolerated than oral airway in pts not deeply unconscious. Caution in pts with severe cranial facial injury		X		X
Endotracheal	Sizes vary - generally larger tubes offer less airway resistance, but should not be so large as to cause damage to vocal cords. See Below for further details.	X	X	X	X
Tracheostomy	Primarily used when Endotracheal Intubation not possible (or contraindicated), or with longer-term mechanical ventilation efforts	X	X	X	X

Endotracheal Tubes (ET Tubes)

Types:

- Regular (with Murphy Eye), usually slightly curved, pliable
- Subglottic tubes (allow for sx above the cuff)
- Anti-Aspiration Designs (microcuff, silver-coated, etc.)

Typical Sizing

	ET Tube I.D.(mm)	Avg Depth	Blade	Mask	Sx Catheter (Fr)
Adult Male	6.5-9.5	21-23	3-4	4	16
Adult Female	6.0-8.5	19-21	3	4	14

Tracheostomy Tubes (Trachs)

Types:

Characteristics	Typical Variations Available
Material	Metal (Jackson) Plastic (Shiley, Portex, Bivona, etc.)
Presence of Cuff	Cuffed or Uncuffed
Type of Cuff	Air, Fluid, or Foam Filled
Shape	Normal versus Speciality (Distal, Proximal, Custom)
Fenestrations	Fenestrated or Unfenestrated
Inner Cannula	None or Removable (Nondisposable, Disposable)
Adjuncts	Speaking Valves (see next page)
Sizes	Vary, Adult usually 4-9

> **!** *A Speaking Valve is a one-way valve (pt can inhale via trach, but then must exhale through upper airway). Cuffed trachs MUST HAVE THE CUFF FULLY DEFLATED when speaking valve is in place.*

Indications for Tracheostomy Placement

- Patients unable to protect their airways
- Excessive secretions
- Failure of noninvasive methods of cough assist
- Swallowing or cough impairment with chronic aspiration
- Patients requiring invasive ventilation > 21 days
- Contraindications to, failed, or cannot tolerate NPPV
- Need to reduce anatomical deadspace for improved oxygenation and/or ventilation

Speaking Valves

Common Brands	• Passy Muir Valve (PMV) • Shiley • Montogomery
Purposes	• Pt Communication • Facilitates swallowing (eating/drinking) • Pt may retain Instrinsic PEEP • Better Secretion Management (cough secretions to upper airway)
Procedure	**DEFLATE TRACH CUFF** • Attach speaking valve to trach • If needed, increase VT on Vent-Dependent pts (leak has been created) • On initial placement, monitor for tolerance: HR, RR, SpO2, WOB, Dyspnea • If indicated, attach O2 to valve
Problems	• Air-trapping • Fatigue • Mucus can occlude one-way valve • Tolerance of Valve

Tracheostomy Troubleshooting Guide

Complication	Possible Causes	Possible Actions
Balloon won't stay inflated	Cuff patent?	Consider Trach Change
Bleeding	Amount in relation to when trach placed/ changed last	Immediately Consult MD
Chest Pain	R/O Cardiac Misplaced Trach Occluded Trach Resp Failure	Request EKG Verify Placement of Trach
Crackling and/ or Edema around stoma	Trach in tissue (sub-q. air)	Immediately consult MD Verify Placement* Consider Trach Change
High Cuff Pressures Should be < 30 mmHg	Incorrect Size?	Consider Trach Change if larger trach due to risk of tracheomalacia over time
Difficulty passing Sx Catheter	Sx Catheter too large? Misplaced Trach? Occluded Trach?	**Consider Lavage. If still unable to pass sx, and/or pt distress, immed. pull trach** If occluded from dried mucus, ensure adequate humidity and sx'ing
Drying of Tracheal Mucosa	Lack of Humidity?	Consider adding Heated (or Cool) Humidity
Excessive Secretions, Change in Secretions	Infection? Lack of Humidity?	Consider Culturing Add Humidity Bronchial Hygiene
Redness of Skin around Tube, Drainage	Infection (may be SOB, febrile)	Consider Culturing Wound Care consult?
Granulation Tissue (immat bld vessels)	Complication of Trach in place for extend. period May Bleed Easily	Consider regular trach changes (1-2 weeks)
Excessive Coughing, Gagging, SOB, Choking	Excessive Secretions Tolerance	Bronchial Hygiene Instill Lidocaine (cautious!) Mech Ventilation?

Replacing a Trach Tube*
(see Important Trach Change Considerations, Next Page)

Inner Cannula

1. Explain procedure to patient
2. Position patient supine or slightly elevated
3. Wash hands vigorously with soap and water
4. Apply gloves
5. Have patient take a deep breath
6. Insert inner cannula gently and lock in place
7. Position pre-cut gauze under trach tube, pulling and set up under ties

Single Tube or Outer Cannula (and accidental extubation)

1. Explain procedure to patient
2. Position patient supine or slightly elevated
3. Wash hands vigorously with soap and water; glove each hand
4. Cleanse surrounding area
5. Remove inner cannula of new tube (if present), insert obturator, and attach new ties. Check new cuff for leaks (if present).
6. Lubricate outside of tube with water-soluble lubricant
7. Oxygenate (if needed), suction trach and upper airway, re-oxygenate. Deflate cuff (if present)
8. Cut ties, have patient take a deep breath (or give deep breath with resuscitation bag), remove old trach tube gently.
9. Quickly, but gently, insert new tube (sideways, then downward) (do not force), hold tube in place and immediately remove obturator.
10. Insert inner cannula and lock in place (if present), inflate cuff, if present.
11. Check for airflow, and observe for difficulty breathing.
12. Remove tube if cannot be placed properly or airflow is inadequate; ventilate as needed and attempt to reinsert tube.
13. Hold tube in place until urge to cough subsides.
14. Secure trach ties (leave one finger width loose).
15. Suction and oxygenate if needed. Auscultate BS.
16. Assess stoma site.
17. Wash hands vigorously with soap and water

* The frequency of tube change depends on airway size, presence of cough, secretion volume and color, malfunction, or grossly dirty or contaminated.

Commonly, adult, cuffed tubes, q 4-8 weeks; uncuffed tubes, q 6 months. Children typically require more frequent changes, due to growth changes.

Tracheostomy Tube Care

Removing and Cleaning Trach Tube

1. Wash hands vigorously with soap and water and apply gloves
2. Open all packages
3. Suction trach tube before removing
4. Remove inner cannula by unlocking/gently pulling outward or remove single tube or outer cannula by cutting ties, holding tube in place with finger, deflate cuff, pull gently outward and downward.
5. Soak tube in cleaning solution for indicated time
6. Clean skin/stoma with cotton dipped in sol. + pat dry with gauze.
7. Brush inside of tube with cleaning solution
8. Rinse tube thoroughly with distilled water
9. Pat dry with clean gauze and replace

Considerations for Trach Changes

Variable	Considerations
Equipment	Always have a BVM at the ready, connected to O_2 with appropriate flow running. Intubation equip. should be easily accessible.
People at Bedside	Per policy, with minimum of one person changing trach and one other qualified medical professional who can assist with airway management
Age of Trach	Fresh tracheostomies (< 1 week old) should be changed only if emergent, and by MD. Risk of loss of patent airway if pulled. Intubation equipment should be present.
Anatomical	**Extreme Caution Should be Used in:** • Obese Patients • Abnormal neck anatomy • Any trach placed for patency (versus ventilation/oxygenation)
Size	Downsizing is generally easier than replacing same size, and extreme caution in upsizing.
Verification	Always verify correct placement following a trach change. Use Auscultation, $ETCO_2$, Chest Rise, Return Volumes if on Vent, SpO_2, WOB, ability to pass sx catheter and/or able to "bag" patient effectively

Stoma Care

- Inspect Stoma site daily for secretions, signs of infection/inflammation (redness), and encrustation (granuloma form.).
- Clean stoma at least daily (more freq if breakdown) with cotton-tipped applicator and water or 1:1 hydrogen peroxide and water or saline solution. Apply Betadine/Polyspirin PRN.
- Change dressing at least once a day
- Trach ties (both velcro and cloth) should be changed as needed. With the flange of the trach tube secured, remove dirty tie and replace with a new, properly sized one, making sure the tie is secure, but not too tight. One finger should fit beneath tie.

Capping and Decannulation

Normal Process of Trach Progression

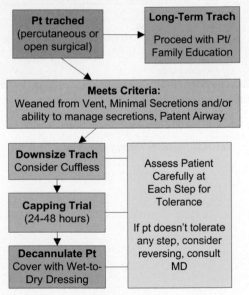

Choosing Humidity Therapy for Patients with Tracheostomies

	Heated Humidifier	Nebulizer	HME-HCH
Efficacy	Good: Efficient, temperature control preferred for long term trach ventil.	Fair: May be too cool, heaters not very practical, may deliver too much water	Fair: Not for thick, copious secretions, marginal humidity, can't use with speaking valves May be used for periods <12 hrs if min secretions
Safety	Fair: May cause burns, electrical hazard, inadvertent lavage from condensation	Fair: Water droplets may cause bronchospasm - del. excess H2O	Fair: No power or condensation hazards, may occlude with secretions, ↑Raw
Cost	Expensive	Fair	Fair
Convenience	Poor: Complex (with heated wire), condensation (w/o heated wire), water refill > 8 hr	Fair: Simple, water refill < 8 hr	Good: Simple, no additional equipment needed

SEE ALSO: Humidity Therapy, this chapter

SEE ALSO: Humidity Therapy, this chapter

Intubation Procedure

Prepare all Equipment, and Fully Assess the Patient prior to intubating:

- Bag and Valve Mask Ventilation (BVM) connected to O2 (12-15 L)
- Laryngoscope (check bulb)
- Blades (Miller or MacIntosh)
- Endotracheal Tube (several sizes), check cuff
  Use new Endotracheal Tube on each Intubation attempt
- 10 cc Syringe
- Stylet (flexible or rigid, depending on intubation apparatus)
- ETCO2 detector, capnography, EDD, etc. for verifying placement

IMPORTANT CONSIDERATIONS:

- Have all possible equipment at bedside to anticipate difficulties (fiberoptic equipment, bronchoscope, etc.)
- Cautious Rapid Sequence Intubation (RSI) in pts who are obese, who are known difficult intubations, etc.
- Pulse Oximetry, Blood Pressure, and EKG must be monitored during intubation. Interrupt attempt if oxygenation/ventilation is needed
- Only direct visualization is completely reliable. Use all possible verification methods. IF IN DOUBT, PULL IT OUT
- Remove tube at once if gurgling in stomach, and no chest expansion

Insertion Distance: Male (21-23 cm); Female (19-21 cm)

Successful Intubation Checklist:

	Lungs: equal + bilateral breath sounds, Chest Expans.
	Abdomen: ↓ sounds in abdom, No ↑ abdom. distention
	Warm air exhaled from ET Tube
	+ ETCO2* (Yellow is YES, Purple is PROBLEM)
	Condensate inside of ET Tube
	Improved pt color/SpO2
	Visualization with Scope
	CXR Verification
	Esophageal Detector Device (EDD)*

End-tidal CO₂ Detector (P$_{ET}$CO₂) for Verification

CO2 Detected	
Tube likely in trachea	May rarely detect CO₂ if tube in esophagus and lg amts of carbonated fluid ingested prior to. This will dissipate after a few ventilations.
CO2 Not Detected	
Tube is in Esophagus	• Absent Chest Rise • Absent Breath Sounds • Stomach gurgling and distension
Tube is in Trachea *Verify with several other methods*	*Decreased CO₂ IN Lungs:* • Poor blood flow to lungs • Cardiac Arrest • Pulmonary Embolus • IV Bolus of Epinephrine *Decreased CO₂ FROM Lungs:* • Airway Obstruct (Status Asthm., etc.) • Pulmonary Edema • Mucus Plugging
Unclear Where Tube Is	Detector Contaminated with gastric contents or acidic drug
ETCO2 device applied incorrectly, Time	Many disposable devices require "activation" (such as by pulling of paper tab), and may req. a few ventilations to change color

Esophageal Detector Device for Verification

Syringe-Type plunger is attached to ET Tube.	
Able to Pull Back on Plunger	ET Tube likely in trachea (rigid structure of trachea allows for air passage)
Unable to Pull Back on Plunger	ET Tube likely in esophagus (floppy structure of esophagus collapses over end of ET tube)

Caution: May be misleading in morbid obesity, late pregnancy, status asthmaticus, or with copious secretions. Use in Children only if > 20 kg with perfusing rhythm.

Management of Airway Emergencies[1]
(AARC CPG)

Indications

Conditions requiring general airway management: airway compromise, protection, respiratory failure.

Conditions requiring emergency tracheal intubation, surgical placement or alternative techniques (see the AARC guideline for a list of numerous specific conditions).

Contraindications

Patient's documented desire not to be resuscitated.

Monitoring

Patient:

Clinical signs – airway obstruction (blood, foreign objects, secretions, vomitus), BS, chest movement, epigastric sounds, LOC, nasal flaring, retractions, skin color, upper airway sounds (snoring, stridor), ventilation ease.

Physiologic variables – ABG, pulse ox., CXR, PeCO2, HR, rhythm, f, VT, Paw.

Tube positioned in trachea:

Confirmed by – chest x-ray, endoscopic visualization, exhaled CO2

Suggested by – BS (bilateral), chest movement (symmetrical), condensate upon exhalation, epigastrium (absence of ventilation sounds), esophageal detector devices, visualization of passage through vocal cords.

Precautions/Hazards/Complications

Emergency Ventilation:

barotrauma, gastric insufflation/rupture, hypo/hyper ventilation, O2 delivery (inadequate), hypotension, unstable cervical spine, upper airway obstruction, ventilation (prolonged interruption), vomiting, aspiration.

Trans-Laryngeal intubation, Cricothyroidotomy:

Aspiration, bronchospasm, laryngospasm, bradycardia, tachycardia, dysrhythmia, hypo/hypertension.

ET tube problems –

Cuff herniation, perforation, extubation (inadvertent), pilot tube valve incompetence, size inappropriate, tube kinking, occlusion.

Failure to establish patient airway, intubate the trachea

Intubation of bronchi, esophagus

Pneumonia

Trauma – airway, cervical spine, dental, esophagus, eye, nasal, needle cricothyroidotomy (bleeding, esophageal perforation, subcutaneous emphysema), vocal cords.

Ulceration, stenosis, malacia

---

1) Adapted from the AARC Clinical Practice Guidelines: Management of Airway Emergencies, *Respiratory Care*, Volume 40, #7, 1995.

Bag and Valve Mask Ventilation (BVM)

Variable	Considerations	
Rates		
	Most Pts	10-12 breaths/min (every 5-6 sec) with 1 sec inspir.
	COPD ↑ Raw Hypovol.	6-8 breaths/min (every 7-10 sec) with 1 sec inspir. - avoids Auto-PEEP -
	CPR	8-10 breaths/min - allows venous return -
Volumes	Estimated (deliver enough for visible chest rise):	
	Adult	500-600 mL (6-7 mL/kg) 1 L Adult Bag: 1/2 - 2/3 vol 2 L Adult Bag: 1/3 vol
	Infant/ Child	Visible Chest Rise Bag size should be > 450-500 mL
Gas Source	Run at 15+ LPM of Oxygen. Verify O_2 flowmeter, and hasn't become disconnected or is on Air	
Personnel	Most effective with 2 Rescuers - 1 opens airway/seals mask, 2nd squeezes bag while both observe chest rise	
Cautions	**Avoid Hyperinflation**	
	Giving > 12 breaths/min (>q 5 sec) may ↑ PIT, ↓venous return, ↓CO, and ↓ coronary and cerebral perfusion.	
	Gastric Inflation	
	Giving large or forceful breaths may cause regurgitation, aspiration, elevated diaphragm, ↓ lung movement, and ↓ CL.	
	Patient Vomits	
	Turn to side, wipe/sx out mouth, return to Supine	
Inadequate Face/Mask Ventilation	• Absent or ↓: bs, chest movement, expired CO_2 • ↓ SpO_2, Cyanosis • Excessive gas leak • Gastric air entry/dilatation • Hemodyn. changes (↑HR, ↑ BP, arrhythmias)	

Suctioning

- Natural coughing is the most desirable method of clearing secretions. Manually assisted coughing or mechanical cough assist (see Lung Expansion Therapy, this Chapter) may reduce the need for suctioning.
- Routine and frequent suctioning is not recommended. Suction catheters traumatize the airway mucosa potentially increasing secretion production, may cause hypoxemia and/or cardiac arrhythmias, possible atelectasis, as well as the risk of infection.
- When suctioning is necessary, perform as gently as possible, keeping the catheter within the tube, if possible.
- If suctioning beyond the tube tip is necessary, the catheter should be advanced gently and suction applied only during catheter withdrawal, with suction being applied for no more than 15 sec.
- Use the lowest suction pressure possible to obtain the desired result. If suction catheter becomes clogged, quickly clear out obstruction, do not increase suction.

Indications/Need

Evidence of Secretions	• Visible secretions in tube • Audible course, wet, +/or ↓ BS • Palpation of wet, course vibrations through chest wall
Alterations in Patient or Ventilation	• Patient: ↑ agitation, irritability, restless • Ventilator: ↑ Raw VV: ↑ PIP and ↑ high pressure alarms PV: ↓ VT
Alterations in Vital Signs	• Change in respiratory pattern: ↑ WOB, tachypnea, retractions • Change in cardiac pattern: ↑ or ↓ HR
Alterations in O₂ and Ventilation	• ↓ SpO₂ (< 90%) • Skin color changes – pale, dusky, or cyanotic • Changes in ABGs - ↑ PaCO₂, ↓ PaO₂, respiratory acidosis

Suction Pressures/Catheter Sizes

Suction Pressures	Suction Catheter Size
Adult -100 to −120 mm Hg Child -80 to −100 mm Hg Infant -60 to −80 mm Hg	ET tube size (ID) x 2, then use next smaller size suction catheter E.g.; 6.0 x 2 = 12, use 10 FR

Suctioning Procedure

1. Assess indications/need as above
2. Set up and test suction pressure (never use "Max")
3. Explain procedure to patient ("this will make you cough")
4. Position patient: (commonly, unless contraindicated)
   Nasaotracheal and pharyngeal suctioning – Semi-Fowler's position with neck hyperextended
   Endotracheal and tracheostomy – supine
5. Wash and glove both hands – use sterile technique
6. Pre-oxygenate with 100% O_2 for 30 sec
7. Note RR, HR, and SpO_2, and monitor throughout procedure
8. Insert catheter as far as possible (until you feel resistance, or until patient begins to cough), then withdraw a few cm. (For ET or trach tubes, advance to just past ET tube tip [shallow sx] or until meet resistance at carina and then withdraw 1 cm [deep sx])
9. Apply suction while withdrawing and rotating the catheter (< 10-15 sec). Do not move catheter up and down. Stop and remove immediately if untoward patient response.
10. Allow patient to rest and reoxygenate for 1 minute
11. Clean secretions from catheter by suctioning sterile water
12. Monitor patient (vital signs and response)
13. Repeat steps 6-11 as needed
14. Return any continuous O_2 to pre-suction settings

NOTES for FOLLOWING PAGE (Nasotracheal Suctioning CPG):

1) The insertion of a suction catheter through the nasal passage and pharynx into the trachea (without a tracheal tube or tracheostomy) to remove material from the trachea and nasopharynx that cannot be removed by the patient's spontaneous cough.
2) Adapted from the AARC Clinical Practice Guideline: Nasotracheal Suctioning, *Respiratory Care*, Volume 37, #8, 1992 and 2004 update.

Nasotracheal Suctioning (2004 Revision & Update)[1,2]
(AARC CPG)

Indications

Patient's cough unable to clear secretions or foreign material in the large central airways.

Evidenced by:

Audible or visible secretions in airway

Chest x-ray (retained secretions → atelectasis or consolidation)

Coarse, gurgling BS or ↓ BS

Hypoxemia or hypercarbia

Suspected aspiration

Tactile fremitus

↑WOB

To stimulate cough or for un-relieved coughing

To obtain sputum sample

Contraindications

Absolute: Croup or epiglottis

Relative: Acute facial, head or neck injury, bronchospasm, coagulopathy or bleeding disorder, high gastric surgery, irritable airway, laryngospasm, MI, nasal bleeding, occluded nasal passages, tracheal surgery, URI.

Pressures

Adult	-100 to -150 mm Hg
Child	-100 to -120 mm Hg
Infant	-80 to -100 mm Hg
Neonate	-60 to -80 mm Hg

Suction time should be < 15 sec.

Frequency

Only when indicated and other measures have failed.

Monitoring

(before, during, and after) BS, cough, CV parameters (HR, BP, EKG), ICP, laryngospasm, oxygen saturation, RR, pattern, SpO2, skin color, sputum (color, volume, consistency, odor), subjective response (pain), trauma, bleeding.

Hazards/Complications

Atelectasis, bronchospasm, CV changes (↓ HR,↑↓BP, arrhythmia, arrest), gagging, vomiting, hypoxia, hypoxemia,↑ ICP (IVH, cerebral edema), laryngospasm, mechanical trauma (bleeding, irritation, laceration, perforation, tracheitis), misdirection of catheter, nosocomial infection, pain, pneumo-thorax, respiratory arrest, uncontrolled coughing.

Assessment of Outcome

Improved BS, improved ABGs or SpO2, secretions removed, ↓WOB (↓RR or dyspnea)

See Notes for this CPG on PREVIOUS PAGE

Airway Clearance Techniques

Variable	Considerations
Indications	**Prevent Secretion Retention** Acute respiratory failure; Atelectasis; Immobile patients; Lung disease (COPD, etc.); Neuromuscular disorders; Post Op? **Remove Copious Secretions** Allergens/irritants; Asthma; Bronchiectasis; Bronchitis; Cystic fibrosis; Infection **Copious Secretions = 25-30 mL/day (1oz/shot glass)**
Signs & Symptoms	**Symptoms** ↑ Chest congestion; ↑ Cough (or ineffective); ↑ SOB or WOB; ↑ Wheezing; ↑ or ↓ Sputum product **Signs** BS – abnormal, audible or ↓; ↑ RR, ↑ HR; ↑ Respiratory tract infections and fever; ↓ SpO2 or worsening ABG's; ↓ Expiratory flow rates; Secretions - ↓ or ↑, thick, or discolored; Chest X-ray changes **Note**: The effectiveness of bronchial hygiene therapy is commonly determined by improvement of the above signs & symptoms
Factors Affecting Secretion Clearance	**Impaired Mucocilliary Transport** Analgesics; Anesthetics; Cigarette smoking; Cuffed ET or trach tube ; Dehydration (dry gases > 4 L/m, bypass of upper airway); Electrolyte imbalance; Hypoxia or hypercapnia; Loss of cilia (COPD, infection); Pollutants **Impaired Cough Force** Abdominal restriction, surgery, pain; Air trapping (emphysema); Airway collapse, constriction, inflammation, obstruction (allergens, asthma, CF, COPD, Infection, irritants, tumors); Artificial airway; CNS depression; Drugs (analgesics/ narcotics); NM weakness, fatigue, paralysis, **Excessive or Thick Secretions** Allergens/irritants; Asthma; Bronchiectasis; Bronchitis; Cystic fibrosis; Infection

Selecting Bronchial Hygiene Therapies

Patient Concerns	Technique Factors
• Ability to self administer is an important factor • Disease type and severity • Fatigue or work required • Pt's age and ability to learn • Patient's pref. and goals	• Clinician skill in teaching the technique • Cost (direct and indirect) • Equipment required • Physician/caregiver goals • Therapy effectiveness

See Bronchial Hygiene Selection Algorithm (pg 10-56) and ACCP Recommendations (pg 10-57)

Make Choices Based Upon the above factors/concerns, but as with most therapies you should consider Least Intense options first, moving to more intense options as a therapy is not effective, or not appropriate for pt clinical condition / ability.

Suggested Order of Therapy Implementation

Least Intense (Self)	• Directed Cough *+ • Diaphragmatic Exercises *+ • Pursed Lip Breathing • Autogenic Drainage/ACBT
(Device)	• Acapella Device • Flutter Valve
Intense (Device + Time)	• Postural Drainage, Percuss. & Vibration*+ • The Vest (and others) *+ • In-Exsufflator (Cough Assist) * • Intrapulmonary Percussive Ventil. (IPV)*+ • Nasotracheal Suctioning (NTS)
Most Intense	• Therapeutic Bronchoscopy * • Intubation (Short-Term) • Tracheostomy (Longer-Term)

* Options for Patients with Non-Vented Patients w/ Artificial Airways
+ Options for Patients who are Mechanically Ventilated

Therapeutic Coughing		
Directed or Therapeutic Coughing		
Indications	May assist in pts with limited cough ability, who are weak/deconditioned, but with adequate neurological function to follow/learn instructions	
Techniques	*Controlled Cough*	Three deep breaths, exhaling normally after the first two and then coughing firmly on the third.
	Double Cough	A deep breath followed by two coughs with the second cough more forceful.
	Three Coughs	A small breath and a fair cough, then a bigger breath and a harder cough, and finally a deep breath with a forceful cough.
	Pump Coughing	A deep breath followed by three short easy coughs, then three huffs.
	Huff Cough (Forced Expiratory Technique [FET])	A slow, deep breath (mid-lung) followed by a 1-3 sec hold, then a series of short, quick, forceful exhalations or "huffs" with the mouth and glottis kept open.
	Manually-Assisted Cough	A deep breath followed by a forceful exhalation, plus an assistant quickly and firmly pushing the abdomen (or lateral costal margins of chest) up against the diaphragm during exhalation. *
Contra-indications	Pregnant women, abdominal pathologies, (e.g., aortic aneurysm, hiatal hernia), and/or unconscious patient with unprotected airways. Lateral costal margin pressure is contraindicated with osteoporosis or flail chest. ACCP does not recommend for patients with airflow obstruction, like COPD.	

Directed Cough[1, 2]
(AARC CPG)

Indications

Atelectasis, post-op prophylaxis, secretion retention/removal, sputum sampling.

Contraindications

Relative: acute unstable head neck or spine injury; ↓coronary artery perfusion (acute MI), inability to control droplet nuclei transmission (TB), ↑ICP, intracranial aneurysm.

Manually assisted cough to epigastrum: abdominal aortic aneurysm, acute abdominal pathology, bleeding diathesis, hiatal hernia, ↑risk of regurgitation/aspiration, pregnancy, untreated pneumothorax.

Manually assisted cough to thorax: flail chest, osteoporosis.

Frequency

PRN, post-op prophylaxis (q 2-4 hrs while awake), during and at end of any bronchial hygiene, FET (as alternative for PDT) (tid, 4 times/day).

Hazards/Complications

Anorexia, vomiting, retching, barotrauma, bronchospasm, central line displacement, chest pain, cough paroxysms, ↓cerebral perfusion, ↓coronary artery perfusion, fatigue, gastroesophageal reflux, headache, incisional pain, evisceration, incontinence, muscle damage/discomfort, paresthesia/numbness, rib or cartilage fracture, vertebral artery dissection, visual disturbance.

Monitoring

Adverse neurologic signs, BS, cardiac arrhythmias, hemodynamic alterations, patient's subjective response (pain, dyspnea, discomfort), pulmonary mechanics (PEF, PEP, PIP, Raw, VC), sputum.

Clinical Goals

Improved: clinical status, subjective response
Sputum production
Stabilized pulmonary hygiene

---

1) A component of any bronchial hygiene therapy when spontaneous cough is inadequate. Includes forced expiratory technique (FET or huff cough) and manually assisted cough.

FET = one or two huffs (forced expiration) from mid to low lung volume with an open glottis (often with brisk abduction of the upper arms), followed by a period of diaphragmatic breathing and relaxation.

Manually assisted cough = external application of mechanical pressure to epigastric region or thoracic cage during forced exhalation.

2) Adapted from AARC Clinical Practice Guideline: Directed Cough, *Respiratory Care*, Vol. 38, #5, 1993.

Active Cycle of Breathing Techniques (ACBT)	
Technique	1. Gentle diaphragmatic breathing at normal VT with relaxation of upper chest and shoulders. 2. Four thoracic expansion exercisees (TEE) - deep inspirations and relaxed expiration 3. Repeat #1 4. Forced Expiration Technique (FET) consists of one or two huffs at appropriate lung volume, dependent on location of secretions, followed ALWAYS by breathing control #1 (e.g. one or two mid- to low-lung volume huffs, if secretions located in more peripheral airways, one or tow high lung volume huffs or cough, if secretions located in larger more central airways followed by #1. 5. Repeat cycle until chest is as clear as possible.
Note	• Avoid cough until secretions for expectoration in upper airways • Intersperse with #1 at any stage, if patient becomes breathless or wheezy

Autogenic Drainage	
Indications	Primarily used for Cystic Fibrosis, though may assist with others with thick secretions. Because of technique required, pt should be > 8 yrs old.
Techniques	• Requires several sessions to learn technique, but is then a self-directed (no equipment) therapy: • Instruct pt to sit or recline, with neck slightly extended. • Three Phases:

	Phase 1 *(Unstick)*	• Inhale small lung volume with a 1-3 sec breath hold • Exhale actively, but not forcefully • Repeat 1-3 minutes until secretions mobilized and heard/ felt in larger middle sized airways (ie, crackles - coarse and loud)
	Phase 2 *(Collect)*	• Inhale medium lung volume with a 1-3 sec breath hold • Exhale actively, but not forcefully • Repeat 1-3 minutes until secretions mobilized and heard/ felt in largest proximal airways (ie crackles - coarser and louder)
	Phase 3 *(Evacuate)*	• Inhale, slow, deep breaths (large lung volumes), with a 1-3 sec breath hold • Exhale actively, more forcefully • Repeat until secretions expectorated with huff or controlled cough • Follow with #1. • Repeat cycle until chest is as clear as possible.

Breathing Exercises

Diaphragmatic Exercises	
Indications	• Alleviate Dyspnea; Improve Oxygenation • Increase Ventilation; Reduce Post-Op Complications
Technique	• Have pt assume comfortable position (sitting supported, semi-fowlers, or supine with hip and knees flexed). • Explain purpose, goals, demonstrate desired result. • Place hand on pt's epigastric area, asking them to breathe slowly and comfortably; follow pt's breathing with hand. • Pursed-lip breathing (as described later in this chapter) is often performed with diaphragmatic breathing. • After several breathing cycles, as the pt completes an exhalation, apply a firm counter-pressure with the hand and ask the patient to inhale and to "fill my hand with air"; observe the expansion under your hand, then instruct pt to exhale normally. • Continue practicing, then have the patient place his or her own hand on their epigastric area and repeat the procedure. • Continue practicing until the pt can perform the exercise properly w/ no verbal cues or having hand on their epigastrium. • As an aid to teaching, the patient may place his other hand over the sternum and instruct the patient to keep that hand from moving up and down. • Advance teaching can be done by having the patient perform the exercise while sitting unsupported, standing, and walking.

Diaphragmatic Strengthening	
Indications	Patients with less than normal diaphragmatic strength
Technique	• The application of progressively increasing manual resistance or weights applied over the epigastric area with the patient in the supine position. • The patient should perform several series of three to five slow sustained deep diaphragmatic breaths with interposed rest periods. • Proper starting weight or pressure should permit full epigastric rise for 15 minutes with no signs of accessory muscle contraction. • Additional weight is added as strength improves.
Note	Positioning the patient in a Trendelenburg position, using the force of abdominal contents to resist the diaphragm, can accomplish the same results. A 15° head down tilt results in approximately 10 lbs. of force against the diaphragm. (Caution when using head-down position, see pg 10-48).

Pursed-Lip Breathing	
Indications	To improve ventilation and oxygenation in patients with air-trapping (Asthma, COPD, etc.)
Technique	• Instruct patient to inhale slowly through the nose • Patient is then told to exhale gently through pursed lips (as though whistling) without any use of abdominal muscles. One part of the breathing cycle should be for inspiration and two parts for exhalation (e.g., 2 sec for TI and 4 sec for TE). • If performed while walking; 2 steps as the patient breathes in and 4 steps as the patient breathes out. E must always be longer than I.

Chest Physiotherapy (CPT)

Postural Drainage (See Diagrams following pages)

Indications	Particularly beneficial in Cystic Fibrosis, May benefit patients with thick, secretions (?)
Technique	• Perform at least 1 hr before or 2 hrs after meals. • Prescribed bronchodilator therapy should be given 15 min before therapy. • Ensure patient loosens any tight or binding clothing. • Drainage should begin with superior segments and progress downward. Lung Segment to be drained should be placed such that main bronchus is pointing ↓ (use of pillows/blankets may assist in positioning) • Maintain position for 3-20 min, depending on quantity and tenacity of secretions and patient tolerance. Limit total treatment time to 30-40 min. • Apoply Percussion and Vibration (see next page) • Have patient cough q 5 min during each position and after therapy (use FET in head down positions). There will be less of a rise in ICP if pt is in upright position during cough.

Monitoring	• Watch for signs of patient intolerance and monitor heart rate, BP, and SpO2 during tx,
	• Signs of respiratory compromise:
	   • ↓ diaphragm excusion in head-down position
	   • Airway obstruction from secretions/collapse
	• ALL THERAPY SHOULD BE ADJUSTED BASED UPON PT'S CLINICAL CONDITION / TOLERANCE

Clinical Notes	• Oxygen requirements may increase during CPT, but should decrease following. Positional changes will alter V/Q and may be either beneficial or detrimental to Oxygenation/Ventilation • **NOTE**: Owing to the potential detrimental side effects and recent evidence showing a beneficial effect of using modified positioning, head-down positioning is no longer recommended to be used with PD&P in neo/peds, by the CF Foundation and various CPG's in Australia, Canada, and Europe. • Controversy still remains about using the head down position in adults. Adults have the ability to voice discomfort and intolerance of a therapy.

Percussion and Vibration	
Indications	Particularly beneficial in Cystic Fibrosis, May benefit patients with thick, secretions (?)
Technique	• Percussion is applied to various lung segments either manually (with cupped hands) or mechanically with a motorized percussor/vibrator type unit (electric or pneumatic). • Chest percussion or clapping and vibration are often used in conjunction with postural drainage. • Percussion or clapping is usually applied for several minutes or as tolerated by the patient. • The therapist should remove rings/jewelry on hands/wrist. • Percussion is followed by vibration on exhalation. • Vibration is applied to the chest area with hands tensing at 6-8 vibrations per second for 4-6 exhalations. • The procedure concludes with a deep cough (several techniques are described in this chapter) and expulsion of secretions. • Patients should be allowed to rest as each lung segment is drained and cleared. • Should not be performed on a bare chest, over heart, stomach, spine, kidneys, women's breasts, chest tubes, incisions, wounds, fractures.

Use is controversial and routine use is not justified. Use may be appropriate in select patients, where PD alone fails to mobilize secretions. See ACCP Recommendations at the end of this section.

Postural Drainage Therapy[1, 2]
(AARC CPG)

Indications

Turning –
Patient unable or unwilling to change positions, ↓ PaO$_2$ associated with position, atelectasis (present or potential), artificial airway present.

Postural drainage –
Secretion clearance difficult: qty > 23-30 mL/day, retained secretions with artificial airway, atelectasis from mucous plugging
Specific diseases: bronchiectasis, cystic fibrosis, cavitating lung disease, foreign body aspiration.

External manipulation of thorax:
additional assistance needed to move secretions
-↑ sputum volume and/or consistency.

Frequency

Turning –
Critically ill and ventilated: q 1-2 hrs
Less acute: q 2 hr

Postural drainage therapy –
Critical care: q 4-6 hrs as indicated
Spontaneous breathing patients: per response to therapy
Re-evaluate frequency order q 48-72 hrs or with change in patient status.

Contraindications

All positions –
Absolute: head and neck injury until stabilized, active hemorrhage with hemodynamic instability.
Relative: BP fistula, empyema, hemoptysis (active), ICP > 20 mm Hg, pleural effusion (large), pulm. edema (CHF), pulm. embolism, rib fracture, spinal injury (acute) or surgery (recent), surg. wound or healing tissue, unable to tol. position.

Trendelenburg position –
Relative: aspiration risk (uncontrolled airway, tube feed or recent meal), distended abdomen, esophageal surg., hemoptysis (recent/gross), uncontrolled hypertension, ICP > 20 mm Hg or any ↑.

Reverse Trendelen. Position
Relative: hypotension, vasoactive medication

External manipul. of thorax-
Relative: bronchospasm, burns, lung contusion, open wounds, osteomyelitis of ribs, osteoporosis, pacemaker (recent transvenous or subcutaneous), chest wall pain, skin grafts (recent) or infections, spinal infusion or anesthesia (recent epidural) subcut. emphysema, TB suspected.

Continued on Next Page

Postural Drainage Therapy
(continued from previous page)

Monitoring	Hazards/Complications
Respiratory parameters (RR, pattern, BS, O₂ Sat, sputum, cough)	Bronchospasm, dysrhythmias, hemorrhage, hypotension, hypoxemia, ↑ ICP, pain or injury, vomit/aspiration.
CV parameters (HR, EKG, BP)	**Clinical Goals**
Skin color, mental function, patient subjective response (pain, discomfort, dyspnea, etc.)	Positive changes in: ABG's, BS, CXR, subjective response, sputum production (↑), ventilator variables (↓Raw, ↑CL), VS.

1) Postural drainage therapy (PDT) is bronchial hygiene therapy with or without percussion and/or vibration, designed to improve mobilization of bronchial secretions, improved V/Q matching, and normalize FRC using gravity and/or external manipulation of the thorax.

2) Adapted from the AARC Clinical Practice Guideline: Postural Drainage Therapy, *Respiratory Care*, Vol. 36, #12, 1991.

External Anatomy of Lungs

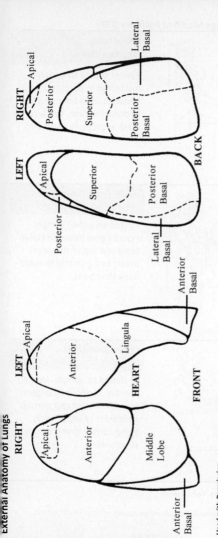

Postural Drainage Modified Positions (CFF)

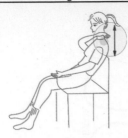

Upper Lobes
(Self Percussion)

Patient should sit upright. Instruct pt to percuss area between collarbone and top of shoulderblade, being careful to avoid bony structures.

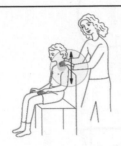

Upper Front Chest

Patient should sit upright. Percuss area between collarbone and top of shoulderblade, being careful to avoid bony structures.

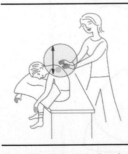

Upper Back Chest

Pt should sit upright, leaning forward at about 30 degrees. Stand behind pt and percuss both sides of upper back, being careful to avoid bony structures.

Used with Permission. Text adapted.

An introduction to postural drainage and percussion. In (2012). Cystic Fibrosis Foundation.

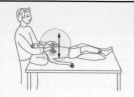

Upper Front Chest

Patient should be supine, with arms to sides. Percuss bilaterally between collarbone and nipple line.

Avoid bony structures and breasts on females.

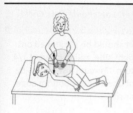

Left Side Front Chest

Patient should be on right side, with left arm over head if able. Percuss over lower ribs, just below nipple line on front of chest.

Avoid abdomen and breasts on females.

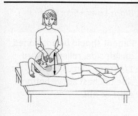

Right Side Front Chest

Patient should be on left side, with right arm over head if able. Percuss over lower ribs, just below nipple line on front of chest.

Avoid abdomen and breasts on females

Used with Permission. Text adapted.

An introduction to postural drainage and percussion. In (2012). Cystic Fibrosis Foundation.

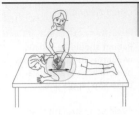

Lower Back Chest

Patient should be proned.
Percuss bilaterally at bottom
of chestwall (use bottom
edge of ribcage as a guide)

Avoid bony stuctures
(lower ribcage and vertebral
column)

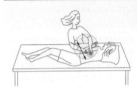

Left Lower Side Back Chest

Pt should be positioned on
right side, rolled forward 1/4
turn. Percuss lower left side
of chest above bottom edge
or ribs

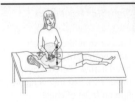

Right Lower Side Back

Patient should be positioned
on left side, rolled forward
1/4 turn. Percuss lower right
side of chest above bottom
edge of ribs

Used with Permission. Text adapted.

An introduction to postural drainage and percussion. In (2012). Cystic Fibrosis
Foundation.

Traditional Postural Drainage Positions

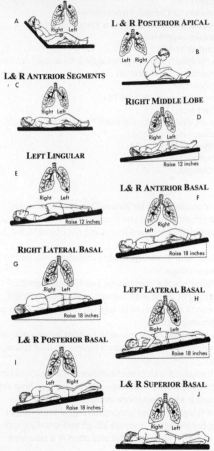

L & R ANTERIOR APICAL

L & R POSTERIOR APICAL

L & R ANTERIOR SEGMENTS

RIGHT MIDDLE LOBE

LEFT LINGULAR

L & R ANTERIOR BASAL

RIGHT LATERAL BASAL

LEFT LATERAL BASAL

L & R POSTERIOR BASAL

L & R SUPERIOR BASAL

Adapted from Hirsch, J. and Hannock, L. *Mosby's Manual of Clinical Nursing Practice.* Copyright 1985 by Mosby.

Potential Effects of a Head-Down Position

- Aggravation of GERD
- Bronchospasm
- Cardiovascular Changes/Hypotension
- Decreased Maximum Expiratory Pressures and PEF
- Decreased oxygenation
- Discomfort or Pain
- Pts with anxiety sometimes struggle with unusual positioning
- Gastrostomy tube aspiration
- Poor tolerance
- Raised Intracranial Pressure (ICP)
- Rib fractures
- Reduced Vital Capacity (Stomach Pressing on diaphragm, impeding lung expansion)
- Shortness of Breath (SOB)
- Uncomfortable
- V/Q Changes

General Considerations for Airway Clearance Techniques

- Most patients breath and cough better when sitting up, leaning slightly forward (head and neck upright, not bent over).
- A pillow held firmly against the abdomen may permit a stronger cough.
- If inspirations are inadequate, teach diaphragmatic breathing or assist with manual bagging or IPPB/NIV.
- Pain medication should be used as prescribed when pain is a limiting factor.
- Patients should be encouraged to drink more water when secretions are extremely thick (unless on fluid restrictions).
- Prior treatment with bronchodilators for bronchospasm, mucolytics/saline/ hypertonic saline may also help aid clearance when secretions are thick and sticky.
- Quadriplegics can use glossopharyngeal breathing or "frog breathing" to improve cough and usually cough better with head of bed flat and often in a side-lying position

In-Exsufflator (Cof-flator™ or Cough Assist™)

Description	Applies a positive pressure to the airway (mask or tube) and then rapidly shifts to a negative pressure producing a high expiratory flow rate from the lungs stimulating a cough.
Indications	The inability to effectively cough or clear secretions as a result of reduced peak expiratory flow rates (< 5-6 L/s) as seen in high spinal cord injuries, neuro-muscular conditions, or fatigue associated with intrinsic lung disorders.
Contraindications	• Bullous emphysema, recent barotrauma, or patients prone to pneumothorax or pneumomediastinum. • Patients with CV instability should be monitored for SpO2 and HR.
Directions for use	• Patients usually given 4 - 5 coughing cycles in succession, followed by a 30 second rest period. • There are usually 6 - 10 cycles for a full treatment. • A typical cycle consists of the following: • The unit slowly builds up positive pressure in the chest over a 1 - 3 sec period to about + 40 mm Hg. • It then rapidly switches to the "exhale" mode with a drop in pressure to – 40 mm Hg in 0.02 seconds (total drop of 80 mm Hg). • Exhalation pressure is usually held for 2-3 sec. • This results in a cough and expectoration of secretions. • The device can be titrated to maximum insufflation by chest wall excursion, BS, and patient comfort. • Some models allow for "Manual" versus "Automatic" modes. In automatic mode, Inspiratory and Expiratory Times and Pressures are set as well as a Pause in between breaths. In Manual Mode, Pressures are set, while timing is via switching from Inspiration to Expiration - Breathing at the same rate with the patient can be helpful in synchronizing. May be used by mouthpiece or mask, as well as by tracheostomy.

Positive Expiratory Pressure (PEP) Therapy	
Description	Positive expiratory pressure (PEP therapy) is the active exhalation against a variable flow resistor reaching pressures of ~ 10-20 cm H_2O.
Indications	PEP Therapy enhances bronchial hygiene therapy by improving airway patency and airflow through airways that are partially obstructed by stenting the airways and/or increasing intrathoracic pressure distal to retained secretions, which: • Reduces air-trapping in susceptible patients • Promotes increased mobilization and clearance of secretions from the airways • Enhances collateral ventilation and opens airways behind mucus obstructions, improving pulm. mech. & facilitating gas exchange Secondarily, it may help prevent or reverse atelectasis, prevent recurrent infection, and slow disease progression.
Devices	Often a disposable, single-patient use device that is self-administered. It is less time-consuming and does not require the precise positioning of chest physical therapy. Used with FET ("huff coughing").
Procedure	1. Instruct to sit upright, with a tight seal around mouthpiece/mask, then inhale, using the diaphragm, to a volume > VT (but not TLC). 2. Instruct to exhale actively, but not forcefully, to FRC, achieving an airway pressure of 10-20 cm H_2O*. I:E ratio 1:3, 1:4 3. Perform 10-20 breaths through the device, then 2-5 huff coughs. 4. Repeat cycle 5-10 times (15-20 minutes) or until secretions are cleared. *The amount of PEP varies with the size of the adjustable orifice and the level of expiratory flow generated by the patient. Adjust to meet patient's need.
Oscillatory PEP	The combination of PEP therapy with airway vibrations or oscillations. See Hig Frequency Oscillations on following pages.

Use of Positive Airway Pressure Adjuncts to Bronchial Hygiene Therapy[1, 2, 3] (AARC CPG)

Indications

Aid in mobilizing secretions (CF, CB)

Optimize bronchodilator delivery

Prevent/reverse atelectasis

Reduce air trapping (asthma, COPD)

Contraindications

Relative: active hemoptysis, acute sinusitis, epistaxis, esophageal surgery, hemodynamic instability, ICP (> 20 mm Hg), middle air problems, nausea, recent surgery (facial, oral, or skull), unable to tolerate (↑WOB), untreated pneumothorax.

Frequency

Critical care: q 1-6 hrs

Acute/domiciliary care: 2-4 x/ day or as needed.

Hazards/Complications

Air swallowing (vomit/aspiration), CV compromise (↓ venous return or ischemia), claustrophobia, ↑ ICP, ↑WOB (hypoventilation /hypercarbia), pulmonary barotrauma, skin breakdown/discomfort.

Monitoring

ABG's/O2 Sat, BS, CV parameters (BP, HR, rhythm), ICP, mental function, RR and pattern, skin color, sputum production (qty, color, consistency, odor), subjective response (pain, dyspnea, discomfort, etc.).

Clinical Goals

↑ sputum production, improved ABG's, BS, chest x-ray, ease of secretion clearance, O2 Sat, &/or vital signs.

---

1) PAP is bronchial hygiene therapy using PEP, EPAP, or CPAP as adjuncts to help mobilize secretions and treat atelectasis.

Positive expiratory pressure (PEP therapy) = exhalation against a fixed orifice resistor reaching pressures of approximately 10-20 cm H_2O.

Expiratory positive airway pressure (EPAP therapy) = exhalation against a threshold resistor reaching preset pressures of 10-20 cm H_2O.

Continuous positive airway pressure (CPAP therapy) = inspiration and expiration within a pressurized circuit and against a threshold resistor maintaining preset pressures of 5-20 cm H_2O.

2) Adapted from the AARC Clinical Practice Guideline: Use of Positive Airway Pressure Adjuncts to Bronchial Hygiene Therapy, *Respiratory Care*, Vol. 38, #5, 1993.

3) Patients should take larger than normal breaths then exhale actively, but not forcefully, creating a positive airway pressure of 10 to 20 cm H_2O. I:E ratio 1:3. Perform 10 - 20 breaths, huff cough 2-3 times, then rest as needed.

Repeat cycle 4-8 times, not to exceed 20 min.

High Frequency Oscillations (HFO) Summary

See Following Pages for Detailed Information on Devices

Airway Oscillations

Patient Generated	*Oscillatory PEP Therapy*	The patient's active exhalation through a device performs the work of creating oscillations which are transferred to the patient's airway.
	Acapella, Flutter, Lung Flute, Quake	
Device Generated	*Intrapulmonary Percussive Ventilation (IPV)*	A device which creates short, rapid inspiratory flow pulses into the airway. Expiration is passive from chest wall elastic recoil.
	MetaNeb, Percussionator, PercussiveNeb, IMP2	

Chest Wall Oscillations

Device Generated	*High Frequency Chest Wall Compression (HFCWC)* *Vest/Cuirass*	A device which creates short, rapid expiratory flow pulses in the airway by compressing the chest wall externally. Chest wall elastic recoil returns lung to FRC.
	The Vest, SmartVest, InCourage	
	High Frequency Chest Wall Oscillation (HFCWO)	A device which creates short, rapid biphasic (positive & negative) pressure changes (oscillations) on the chest wall externally, which is transferred to the airway.
	Hayek Oscillator	

Acapella™	
Description	A disposable, single-patient use device (self-administered) that delivers positive expiratory pressure with high frequency oscillations. Vibratory positive Expiratory Pressure Therapy
Directions	Pt exhales air through an opening that is periodically closed by a pivoting cone. As air passes through the opening, the cone will open and close the airflow path. This produces a vibratory pressure waveform - allowing secretions to be mobilized and expectorated.
Settings	Dial on end of device sets vibration/oscillation frequency (6-20 Hz). Device is available in three flow rate ranges.

Flutter Device™	
Description	A device which produces oscillations in expiratory pressure and airflow. The resultant vibration of the airways loosens mucus from the airway walls.
Contraindications	Patients with Pneumothorax or Right Heart Failure
Directions	• Patient seated with back straight, head tilted slightly back or seated with elbows resting on a table with head tilted slightly back. • Initially, stem is positioned horizontally. Then adjusted up or down to get the maximum "fluttering" effect within the patient's chest (Vibrations can be felt by placing one hand on back and the other on the front of chest). • Patient takes a deep breath (but not to TLC), holds for 2-3 seconds, then exhales actively (but not forcefully) as long as possible while keeping cheeks as hard and flat as possible. • Exhale repeatedly through the device until coughing is stimulated. • Continue for approx. 15 minutes or until patient feels no additional mucus can be raised. • Perform procedure 2-4 times/day or as directed.

Intrapulmonary Percussive Ventilation™ (IPV)	
Description	The delivery of high-frequency percussive breaths (sub-tidal volume) into the patient's airways by a pneumatic device.
Indications	The inability to effectively cough or clear secretions as a result of reduced peak expiratory flow rates.
Contra-indications	Bronchospasm, lung contusion, pneumothorax, pulmonary hemorrhage, subcutaneous emphysema, TB, vomiting and aspiration.
Directions	• Pt breathes through a mouthpiece or artificial airway and the unit delivers high flow rate bursts of gas into the lungs from 100-300 x/min. Continuous positive pressure is maintained (typically 15-40 cm H2O) while the pulses dilate the airways. At the end of the percussive inspiratory cycle (5-10 sec), a deep exhalation is performed with expectoration of secretions. • Normal treatment time is 20 min. Aerosols (Bland or Medicated) may also be delivered via the attached nebulizer with this therapy.
Settings	• Pressure is set via a manometer with optimum range being 30-40 cmH2O (less for ↑ Compliance, more for ↓ Compliance). This is equivalent to setting a "Mean Airway Pressure" • Difficulty knob changes the frequency of the oscillations, which may improve clearance and recruitment. It is recommended that this knob be turned back and forth every few minutes during tx.
Notes	• This therapy can be done as an adjunct to Mechanical Ventilation • Very Important: Circuit configurations are different for ventilator versus non-vented, and should be assembled carefully • When effective, several breaks may need to be taken in order to get pt to cough or suction. • Many clinicians recommend utilizing an inline suction catheter when used in conjunction with an artificial airway to facilitate suctioning. • Cuffed artificial airways: Sx above cuff, and then at least partially deflate cuff during tx to facilitate secretion clearance.

Vest Airway Clearance System™

Description	• The system includes an air pulse generator, inflatable vest, and connecting tube. • It provides high frequency chest wall compressions which help mobilize secretions.
Indications	• Follow the guidelines established by the AARC for airway clearance therapies. • A patient-specific assessment should always be used weighing potential benefits and risks. • Indications include cystic fibrosis, bronchiectasis, or conditions where the patient has the inability to effectively mobilize and expectorate secretions.
Contra-indications	Active hemorrhage, cardiac instability, chest wall pain, lung contusion, recent thoracic skin grafts, recently placed pacemaker, subQ emphysema, suspected TB, unstabilized head and/or neck injury.
Directions	• As the patient wears the inflatable vest, small gas volumes alternately flow into and out of the unit – rapidly inflating and deflating (compressing and releasing) the chest wall to create air flow and cough- like shear forces to move secretions. • Timing of the pulse is manually controlled by the patient or clinician • The intensity (25-40 mm Hg) and frequency (5-25 Hz) of the pulses can also be adjusted by the patient or clinician • Vests come in various styles (full chest vest down to simple wrap around chest), disposable/nondisposable, and sizes. Ensuring a proper fit and style helps ensure better pt compliance with therapy.

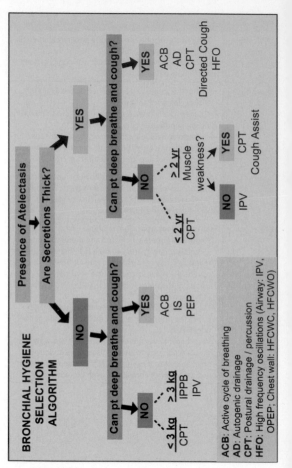

BRONCHIAL HYGIENE SELECTION ALGORITHM

Presence of Atelectasis

Are Secretions Thick?

NO

Can pt deep breathe and cough?

YES — ACB, IS, PEP

NO
- ≤ 3 kg — CPT
- ≥ 3 kg — IPPB, IPV

YES

Can pt deep breathe and cough?

YES — ACB, AD, CPT, Directed Cough, HFO

NO
- < 2 yr — CPT
- ≥ 2 yr — Muscle weakness?
  - YES — CPT, Cough Assist
  - NO — IPV

ACB: Active cycle of breathing
AD: Autogenic drainage
CPT: Postural drainage / percussion
HFO: High frequency oscillations (Airway: IPV, OPEP; Chest wall: HFCWC, HFCWO)

Adapted from:

Chatburn, RL: High Frequency Assisted Airway Clearance. *Respiratory Care*, 2007 52 (9): 1232

Wilkins, RL, et.al: *Egan's Fundamentals of Respiratory Care*, 9th Ed, 2008, pgs918 & 942, Mosby.

Summary Recommendations by the ACCP*

Autogenic Drainage

Should be taught as an adjunct to postural drainage for patients with CF . . . can be performed without assistance and in one position.

Chest Physical Therapy

Recommended in CF patients as an effective technique to increase mucus clearance. The effects of each treatment are relatively modest and the long-term benefits are unproven.

Cough Assist

Mechanical cough assist devices are recommended in pts with NM disease w/ impaired cough, prevents respiratory complications.

Expiratory Muscle Training

Recommended in patients with NM weakness and impaired cough, to improve peak exp. pressure, which may benefit cough.

High Frequency Techniques

Devices designed to oscillate gas in the airway, either directly or by compressing the chest wall, can be considered as an alternative to chest physiotherapy for patients with CF.

Huff Cough

Huff coughing should be taught as an adjunct to other methods of sputum clearance in patients with COPD and CF.

Manually-Assisted Cough

Should be considered in patients with expiratory muscle weakness to reduce the incidence of respiratory complications. Manually assisted cough may be detrimental and should not be used in persons with airflow obstruction caused by disorders like COPD.

Positive Expiratory Pressure Therapy

Recommended in patients with CF over conventional chest physio-therapy, because it is approximately as effective as chest physiotherapy, and is inexpensive, safe, and can be self-administered.

"The effect of nonpharmacologic airway clearance techniques on long-term outcomes such as health-related quality of life and rates of exacerbations, hospitalizations, and mortality is not known at this time."

* Nonpharmacologic Airway Clearance Therapies: ACCP Evidence-Based Clinical Practice Guidelines, *Chest*. 2006; 129:250S-259S.

Additional Resources

See Oakes' **RespiratoryUpdate.com** for further information and explanations of Airway Clearance Techniques, including direct links to:

Evidence-Based Guidelines
- Airway Clearance Techniques (CFF)
- Nonpharmacologic Airway Clearance Therapies (ACCP)
- Use of Positive Airway Pressure Adjuncts to Bronchial Hygiene Therapy (AARC)

Journal Articles and Teachings to include:
- Airway Clearance: Physiology, Pharmacology, Techniques, and Practice
- Autogenic Drainage
- High-Frequency External Chest Wall Compression
- And more

RESPIRATORY UPDATE

THE Virtual Critical Care Library

Humidity Therapy

Variable	Considerations
Indications	**Primary Indications** • Humidify dry medical gases (>4 L/m) • Overcome humidity deficit when upper airway is bypassed **Secondary Indications** • Treat bronchospasm due to cold air • Treat hypothermia • Thickened secretions
Therapeutic Modalities	Used specifically with the following modalities: • Oxygen therapy (esp. when >4 L/m is delivered) • Non-invasive positive pressure ventilation (CPAP and BiPAP ventilation) • Invasive positive pressure ventilation • Artificial Airways via collar or T-Piece
Under-Humidification	• Atelectasis (mucus plugging) • Dry, nonproductive cough • Subsernal pain • Thick, dehydrated secretions • Hypoxemia • ↑ Airway Resistance • ↑ Infection • ↑ WOB
Over-Humidification	• Fluid overload • Pulmonary edema • Surfactant alteration • Thermal damage to mucosa • ↑ Airway secretions (↑ airway resistance) • Atelectasis • Hypoxemia
Heat	• Heated Humidification is recommended for artificial airways, thick secretions, and/or patient comfort

Humidification Devices

Type	Use	Comments
Low Flow		
Bubble Diffuser	Used with low flow devices (>4 L/m) and AEM masks (> 50%)	Provides only 20% to 40% of body humidity, may be heated to deliver 100% humidity (and with low flows >7 L/m), should not be used for patients with ET tube or tracheostomy.
High Flow		
Cascade Humidifier	Mainstream "bubble" humidifier for patients with ET tube or tracheostomy.	100% humidity and body temperature Correct water level is required.
Passover Humidifier	Used for either low or high flow devices (CPAP/ BiPAP) and ventilators.	Effective humidity only when heated to body humidity.
Wick Humidifier	Mainstream "passover" using a porous hygroscopic "wick" to ↑ surface area.	100% humidity and body temperature.
Heat/Moisture Exchanger (HME) (Hygroscopic condenser humidifier [HCH] or artificial nose)	Mainstream "passover" reservoir containing hygroscopic material. Short-term use only with MV (≤ 5 days) *Additional info can be found in Oakes' Mechanical Ventilation Pocket Guide.	Condenses and "traps" exhaled heat and moisture and then evaporates and warms and humidifiers (≈ 70% BH) the inhaled gas. Exchange daily or per manufacturer's recommendations -- Monitor sputum viscosity.
Room Humidifier (cool mist, steam vaporizer, centrifugal)	Used to humidify the room.	Produces 100% humidity at room temperature when in a closed area. Should not be used with ET tube or trach.

Notes (from opposite page):

Distilled or sterile water should be used in bubble humidifiers.
Monitor patient's quantity and quality of airway secretions.

HME: Inspect regularly for partial or complete obstruction by secretions, especially useful during transporting or weaning MV patients.

Heated Humidifier

- Close monitoring of operating and output temperatures, adequate water supply/proper level, and condensation buildup is required.
- Prevent inadvertent tracheal lavage from the condensate.
- Check that alarms are set and working properly
- Choosing Humidity Therapy for Patients with Tracheostomies – See page 10-29

Humidification during Mechanical Ventilation[1]
(AARC CPG)

Indication
Continuous gas therapy: high flow or bypassed upper airway.

Contraindication
None except HME when:
Body temperature < 32°C, concurrent aerosol therapy, expired V_T < 70% of delivered V_T, spont $\dot{V}_E$ > 10 L/min, thick, copious, or bloody secretions.

Monitoring
Check: alarm settings (30 – 37°C) (HR), humidifier temp setting (HR), inspired gas temp (33 ± 2°C) (HR), water level and feed system (HR), sputum quantity and consistency
Remove condensate in circuit
Replace HMEs contaminated with secretions

Frequency:
Continuous during gas therapy

Hazards/Complications
Burns (patient or caregiver)(HR)
Electrical shock (HR)
Hypo/hyperthermia
Hypoventilation (HME → ↑VD)
↑ Resistive WOB through humidifier
Infection (nosocomial)
Tracheal lavage (pooled condensate or overfilling) (HR)
Underhydration (mucous impaction or plugging of airways → air-trapping, hypoventilation, ↑ WOB)
Ventilator malperformance: pooled condensate → ↑ airway pressures or asynchrony with patient (HR)
HME → ineffective low pressure alarm during disconnection

Clinical Goal
Humidified and warmed inspired gases without hazards or complications.

1) Adapted from AARC Clinical Practice Guideline: Humidification during Mechanical Ventilation, *Respiratory Care*, Vol. 37, #8, 1992.
HR = heated reservoir, HME = heat moisture exchanger

Lung Expansion Therapy

Variable	Considerations	
Indications	Risk for, or evidence of Atelectasis (usually secondary to pt either not taking deep breaths, or unable to)	
	Passive Atelectasis	Persistent use of small Tidal Volumes (anesthesia, rib fx, drugs, fatigue, immobilitiy, NM disorders, pain, surgery)
	Resorptive Atelectasis	Ventilation blocked by foreign body, mucus plugs, lesion, or spasm
Clinical Signs	• **History:** • Recent abdominal or thoracic surgery • COPD or cigarette smoking • Prolonged bed rest • Morbid Obesity • **↑ RR, ↑ HR** • **Auscultation:** • Crackles (fine) • Bronchial (consolidation) • ↓ BS (blocked airways) • **CXR:** • ↓ volumes • Opacity • Air bronchograms • Elevated diaphragm • Tracheal shift (severe)	

Minimally Intensive (Self)	• Encourage Deep Breaths
(Device)	• Incentive Spirometry • PEP Therapies (Acapella, Flutter) - see Airway Clearance Section
Intensive (Device + Time)	• Intermittent Pos Pressure Breathing (IPPB) • Intrapercussive Ventilation (IPV) - see Airway Clearance Section • Continuous Positive Airway Pressure (CPAP)
Most Inten	• Therapeutic Bronchoscopy (resorptive)

Incentive Spirometry (IS)	
Description	• Device which encourages deep breathing, usually with measurement (mL) of breath size, as well as indicator of speed (slow is more effective)
Technique	• Designed to mimic natural sigh breaths, by encouraging patients to take slow, deep diaphragmatic inspirations (performing an IC from FRC to near TLC), followed by 5-10 sec breath hold. • Pt should be sitting upright to be most effective. • Directions should be intentionally worded (put the mouthpiece in your mouth, and then take a slow deep breath like you're drinking a milkshake from a straw). Demonstration may assist in learning. • Set realistic goals, but ones that encourage pt to keep pushing further. • Patient should exhale normally and then rest as long as necessary between maneuvers (prevents resp alkalosis) • Each session should contain a minimum of 5-10 breaths, generally with a minimum of 10 breaths/hour.
Notes	• For post-surgical use, it is best to teach technique prior to surgery and have pt practice (it is more difficult to teach a new skill with pain medication interfering). • Device should be placed in plain sight and reach of pt. Instruct family and/or other available staff to assist in encouraging compliance. • For pts that struggle with technique/coordination, consider instead on focusing on key elements without device - deep, slow breaths with 5-10 second hold.

Incentive Spirometry[1, 2]
(AARC CPG)

Indications

Screen at-risk pts for Post-Op Complications:
Preop screening to obtain baseline*
Atelectasis or predisp. for*:
Surgery (upper/lower abdom, thoracic, COPD, prolonged bedrest, lack of pain control, restrictive lung defect (dysfunctional diaphragm or muscles, NM disease, SCI), sickle cell, CABG
*See also recommendations below

Contraindications

Patient unable or unwilling to use device appropriately (including young pts, delirium, heavy sedation)
Patient unable to take deep breath (VC < 10 mL/kg or IC < 1/3 predicted)

Hazards/Complications

Fatigue
Hyperventilation
Inappropriate (as sole tx for major collapse/consolidat)
Ineffective (if used incorrectly)
Hypoxemia (O2 therapy interrupt)
Pain

Monitoring

Initial instruction and observation of proper performance.
Periodic observation for:
compliance, frequency, number of breaths/session, volume or flow goals (improvement), effort, motivation, device availability,

Suggested Frequencies

10 breaths q. 1-2 hr - awake
10 breaths - 5x/day
15 breaths q. 4 hrs

Outcome Assessment

Decreased atelectasis –
BS improved, fever resolved, ↑oxygenation, reduced FIO2 requirement, improved chest x-ray, pulse rate normal, respiratory rate ↓

See Next Page for Evidence-Based Recommendations
(based on GRADE scoring system)

---

1) IS is a component of bronchial hygiene therapy designed to encourage spontaneous breathing patients to take long, slow, deep breaths and hold them for ≥3 seconds (sustained maximal inspiration, SMI). The primary purpose is to help maintain airway patency and prevent/reverse atelectasis.

2) Adapted from the AARC Clinical Practice Guideline: Incentive Spirometry, *Respiratory Care*, Volume 56, #10, 2011.

AARC Evidence-Based Recommendations: IS
 (based on GRADE system)

- Incentive spirometry alone is **not** recommended for routine use in the preoperative and postoperative setting to prevent postoperative pulmonary complications.
- It **is** recommended that incentive spirometry be used with deep breathing techniques, directed coughing, early mobilization, and optimal analgesia to prevent postoperative pulmonary complications.
- It **is** suggested that deep breathing exercises provide the same benefit as incentive spirometry in the preoperative and postoperative setting to prevent postoperative complications
- Routine use of incentive spirometry to prevent atelectasis in patients after upper-abdominal surgery is **not** recommended
- Routine use of incentive spirometry to prevent atelectasis after coronary artery bypass graft surgery is **not** recommended.
- It **is** suggested that a volume-oriented device be selected as an incentive spirometry device.

Intermittent Positive Pressure Breathing (IPPB)		
Goal	• An augmented VT, achieved with min. effort	
Technique	• A semi-Fowler's position is preferred; supine is acceptable when an upright position is contraindicated. • Effectiveness is usually dependent on proper patient instruction and demonstration. • Use mouthpiece/noseclips - mask as last resort. • Optimal breathing pattern is slow, deep breaths held at end-inspiration. • Resulting volumes should be measured and pressure adjusted according to needs and response. • Note: To be effective, Deliv VT > Pt spont efforts • Bland aerosols (NSS) can be delivered via IPPB, but more often, medicated aerosols consisting of a bronchodilator, mucoactive or combination are used. • Treatments usually last 15 - 20 minutes.	
Common Goals and Settings	Parameter	Suggested Goal/Setting
	Sensitivity	1-2 cmH$_2$O (easy trigger, but no autocycle)
	Pressure	Initial: 10-15 cmH2O Goal: set to Target VT (see below)
	Target Vol.	10-15 cc/kg PBW (30% pred. IC)
	Rate	6 breaths/min
	I:E Ratio	1:3 to 1:4
Trouble-shooting	Large negative Pressure swings	Incorrect sensitivity: set to autotrigger, then decrease sens until pt able to trigger easily
	↓ Press after insp. begins, or failure to rise until breath's end	Inspiratory flow too low
	Premature cycle off	Insp flow too high or airflow obstructed (kinked tubing, occluded mouthpiece, active resistance to inhalation)
	Failure to cycle off	Leak (neb, exhalation, pt interface, nose)

IPPB[1, 2]
(AARC CPG)

Indications
Lung expansion –
Atelectasis (when not responsive to other therapies or patient can't/won't cooperate)
Secretions (inability to clear)
Short-term ventilation (alternative form of MV for hypoventilating patients, consider NPPV)
Delivery of aerosolized medication [3] –
Used when other aerosol techniques have been unsuccessful. [4]
Patients with fatigue, severe hyperinflation or during short-term ventilation.

Assessment of Need
Acute, severe, unresponsive bronchospasm/ COPD exac.
Impending respiratory failure NM disorders
PFT (FEV1 < 65% pred, FVC < 70% pred, MVV < 50% pred, VC < 10 mL/kg) w/o eff cough
Significant atelectasis

Contraindications
Absolute – untreated tension pneumothorax
Relative – active hemoptysis, active untreated TB, air swallowing, bleb, hemo instability, hiccups, ICP > 15 mm Hg, nausea, recent oral, facial, esophageal or skull surgery, TE fistula.

Monitoring
Patient: RR, V_T, HR, rhythm, BP, BS, response (mental function, pain, discomfort, dyspnea), skin color, O_2 Sat, sputum, ICP, chest x-ray.
Machine: f, V_T peak, plateau, PEEP pressures, sensitivity, flow, FIO_2, T_I, T_E.

Clinical Goals
For lung expansion: a V_T of at least 33% of IC predicted
↑ FEV_1 or PF
More effective cough, enhanced secretion clearance, improved chest x-ray and BS, good patient response.

Hazards/Complications
Air trapping (auto PEEP), barotrauma, ↓venous return, exacerbation of hypoxemia, gastric distention, hemoptysis, hyperoxia (with O_2), hypocarbia, hypo / hyperventilation, ↑Raw, V/Q mismatch, infection, psychological dependence, secretion impaction.

Frequency
Critical care: q 1-6 hrs as tolerated, re-evaluate daily

Acute care: bid to 4 times per day per patient response, re-evaluate q 24 hrs

SEE NOTES NEXT PAGE

NOTES (from Previous Page)

1) Intermittent positive pressure breathing (IPPB) is intermittent, or short-term mechanical ventilation for the purpose of augmenting lung expansion, assisting ventilation, and/or delivering an aerosolized medication (not the therapy of first choice) (Does not include NPPV).

2) Adapted from the AARC Clinical Practice Guideline: IPPB, 2003 Revision + Update, *Respiratory Care*, Volume 48, #5, 2003.

3) Efficacy is technique dependent (coordination, breathing pattern, VI, PIP, inspiratory hold), device design, and patient instruction.

4) MDI or nebs are devices of choice for aerosol therapy to COPD or stable asthma patients.

Cylinder Color Standards, by Gas

Gas	USA	ISO*
Oxygen (O$_2$)	GREEN	WHITE
Air	YELLOW/SILVER	WHITE/BLACK
Carbon dioxide (CO$_2$)	GRAY	GRAY
CO$_2$ and O$_2$	GRAY/GREEN	GRAY/WHITE
Helium (He)	BROWN	BROWN
He and O$_2$	BROWN/GREEN	BROWN/WHITE
Nitrous Oxide (N$_2$O)	BLUE	BLUE
Cyclopropane (C$_3$H$_6$)	ORANGE	ORANGE
Ethylene (C$_2$H$_4$)	RED	VIOLET
Nitrogen	BLACK	BLACK

*ISO: International Standards Organization

SEE ALSO:

Oxygen Blending Ratios	See pg 9-28
Oxygen Entrainment Ratios	see pg 9-30
Oxygen Duration Times	see pg 9-29
Oxygen Assessment Equations	see pg 9-4

E-Cylinder (O₂) Estimated Tank Duration in Minutes
(0.28 x PSI / LPM)

LPM	Pressure (PSI)							
	500 (reserve)	750	1,000	1,250	1,500	1,750	2,000	2,200
1	140	210	280	350	420	490	560	616
2	70	105	140	175	210	245	280	308
3	46	70	93	116	140	163	186	205
4	35	52	70	87	105	122	140	154
5	28	42	56	70	84	98	112	123
6	23	35	46	58	70	81	93	102
10	14	21	28	35	42	49	56	61
12	11	17	23	29	35	40	46	51
15	09	14	18	23	28	32	37	41

H-Cylinder (O₂) Estimated Tank Duration in Minutes
(3.14 x PSI/LPM)

LPM	Pressure (PSI)							
	500 (reserve)	750	1,000	1,250	1,500	1,750	2,000	2,200
1	1570	2355	3140	3925	4710	5495	6280	6908
2	785	1177	1570	1962	2355	2747	3140	3454
3	523	785	1046	1308	1570	1831	2093	2302
4	392	588	785	981	1177	1373	1570	1727
5	314	471	628	785	942	1099	1256	1381
6	261	392	523	654	785	915	1046	1151
10	157	235	314	392	471	549	628	690
12	130	196	261	327	392	457	523	575
15	104	157	209	261	314	366	418	460

*These charts represent total duration with no Reserve. Best Clinical practice dictates not including the last 500 PSI in your calculation (this is emergency reserve). In order

See Chapter 9 for Detailed Oxygen Duration Equations

Oxygen Monitoring

Method	Normal Values	Description
Noninvasive		
SpO_2	> 95%	Peripheral O_2 saturation (measured Hb saturation via Pulse Oximeter)
TCM	~80-100 mmHg	Transcutaneous Monitoring estimates PaO_2 by inducing hyperperfusion (via heating) of skin site, and measures electrochemically
Invasive		
PaO_2	80 -100 mmHg	Partial Pressure of Oxygen molecules within blood (not those bound to hemoglobin)
SaO_2	95-95%	Calculated O_2 saturation from PaO_2 (if an analysis), or actual measured value (co-oximeter)

Notes:

- Trends are more important than absolute values.
- SpO_2 may be a poor indicator of SaO_2
- Periodic baseline correlations should be made with PaO_2 and/or SaO_2 (CO-oximetry).
- Pulse oximetry alone can not indicate hyperoxemia (maximum is 100%).
- SpO_2 values may vary between various models of oximeters, so caution in interchanging oximeters on same pt
- Factors affecting SpO_2 – See AARC CPG, see Next Page

Noninvasive Monitoring

See following pages

Pulse Oximetry[1,2]
(AARC CPG)

Indications
Need to monitor SaO_2, need to quantitate patient's response to therapy or diagnostic procedure.

Contraindications
Ongoing need to measure pH, $PaCO_2$, total Hgb, and or abnormal Hgb (relative).

Hazards/Complications
Inappropriate therapy due to false negative or positive results, probe misuse (pressure sores, burns, electrical shock).

Frequency
Variable depending on clinical status, indications, and procedures being performed.

Monitoring
Validity of reading –
Compare SpO_2 with SaO_2 and HR with pulse rate (initial and periodic).
Document conditions: patient position, activity level, assess site perfusion, probe location, type of oxygen therapy.
Check for invalidating factors: abnormal Hgb, exposure to light, hyperoxemia, intravascular dyes, low perfusion state, motion artifact, nail polish/covering, saturation < 83%, skin pigmentation.

Patient – vital signs

Clinical Goal
(desired outcome)
To reflect the patient's clinical, oxygenation, condition.

[1] Pulse oximetry (SpO_2) is a noninvasive determination of oxyhemoglobin saturation (SaO_2).

[2] Adapted from the AARC Clinical Practice Guideline: Pulse Oximetry, *Respiratory Care*, Vol. 36, #12, 1991

! Pulse oximetry is helpful in identifying changes in lung function and establishing the need for a change in or discontinuation of O_2 therapy.

The Respiratory Care Practitioner must be acutely aware of the potential inaccuracies of oximetry readings and take them into account when recommending changes. Never use oximetry results as the only parameter when making respiratory care decisions.

Troubleshooting the Pulse Oximeter

Problem	Possible Cause(s)	Interventions
Inaccurate SpO$_2$ (does not correlate with SaO2 from ABG)	**Patient**	
	• Movement • Poor perfusion (cool skin, PVD, etc.) • Skin pigment (darker) • High carboxyhemoglobin or methemoglobin • Reduced arterial blood flow	• Encourage pt to be still, if possible or able • Check sensor site - consider moving from one finger to another, earlobe, toe, forehead, nare • Consider replacing sensor • Use other forms of measure if needed to confirm (ABG, TCM, etc.) • Warm site with approved warming device
	Environment	
	• Cool Room • Ambient Light • BP Cuff Placement	• Warm site with approved warming device • Cover sensor to block ambient light • Ensure sensor is not distal to BP cuff
	Equipment	
	• Blood Pressure • Sensor not adhering well	• Ensure sensor is placed securely; replace if necessary. • Check sensor site - consider moving from one finger to another, earlobe, toe, forehead, nare • Consider different type of sensor (neonatal, etc.) • Use ECG signal synchronization. • Select a longer (10-15 sec) averaging time, if possible.

Problem	Possible Cause(s)	Interventions
Loss of Pulse Signal, Poor Waveform	**Patient**	
	• Reduced arterial blood flow	• Confirm or follow with ABG
	• Anemia	• Check Hemoglobin level
	• Hypothermia	• Consider warming site, replace sensor
	• Shock (hypotension, vasocon)	• Always check pt's condition, Vitals
	• Nail polish	• More likely to intefere if contains metallic flakes, remove
	Environment	
	• Excessive ambient light	• Cover sensor to block ambient light
	Equipment	
	• Constriction by sensor	• Check sensor
	• Sensor is not on patient	• Move to a different site or change type of sensor used
		• Confirm sensor is on patient
Inaccurate Pulse Rate	**Patient**	
	• Excessive patient motion	• Encourage pt to be still if possible, or able
	Equipment	
	• Pronounced dicrotic notch on art. waveform	• Move sensor to a different site
	• Poor quality ECG signal	• Check ECG leads; replace if necessary.
	• Electrocautery interference	• Same as above.

10-74

Arterial Puncture – See AARC CPG: Sampling for Arterial Blood Gas Analysis, Chapter 2

Arterial Line – See Oakes' Hemodynamic Monitoring: A Bedside Reference Manual for an excellent review of indications, insertion sites, equipment, insertion techniques, maintenance, infection control, drawing a blood sample, pressure and waveform variations, complications, trouble-shooting, and removal of the A-Line.

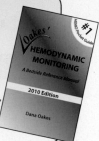

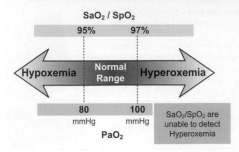

Normal Variations:

Due to FIO_2, barometric pressure, or age

$$(PaO_2 \approx 110 - \tfrac{1}{2} \text{ patient's age})$$

SaO_2 = Calculated O_2 saturation from PaO_2 (if an analysis)
(actual measured value if with a co-oximeter)

SpO_2 = Peripheral O_2 saturation (measured value of Hb saturation
with a pulse oximeter).

PaO2-SaO2 Relationship

PaO_2	SaO_2*
150	100 %
100	97 %
80	95 %
60	90 %
55	88 %
40	75 %

*varies with shifts in oxyhemoglobin curve

!

**Always Check for
Proper Correlation between the
PaO2/SaO2 calculated values and
the measured SpO2 value.**

Factors affecting SaO_2 and/or SpO_2 readings - See AARC
Clinical Practice Guideline

Oxyhemoglobin Dissociation Curve

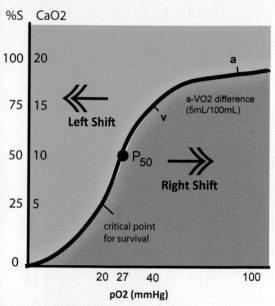

Curve shift = the Bohr effect

a = normal arterial blood

v = normal venous blood

P₅₀ = PaO₂ @ 50% Saturation (normal = 27 mmHg)

Left Shift (↑ Hgb-O₂ affinity; ↓ P₅₀)	Right Shift (↓ Hgb-O₂ affinity; ↑ P₅₀)
Alkalosis Decreased: temp, PCO₂, PO⁴, 2,3 DPG (stored blood) Polycythemia Abnormal Hgb (Fetal Hgb, HgbCo, metHgb)	Acidosis Increased: temp, PCO₂, PO⁴, 2,3 DPG Anemias (sickle cell) Chronic hypoxemia (high altitude)

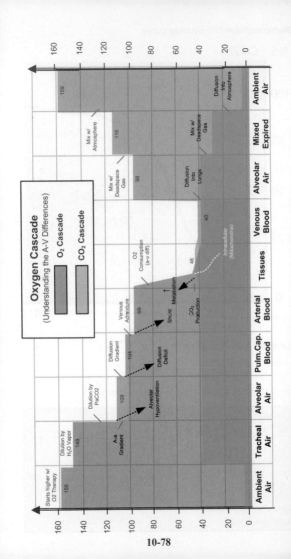

10-78

Assessment of Oxygenation

Oxygenation at the Lungs (external respiration)			Oxygenation at the Tissues (internal respiration)		
	Norm	Ab-norm		Norm	Ab-norm
Adequacy					
PaO_2*	80-100 mmHg	< 80 mmHg	$P\bar{V}O_2$	35-42 mmHg	< 35 or > 45 mmHg
CaO_2	15-24 mL/dL	↑↓	$C\bar{V}O_2$	12-15 mL/dL	↑↓
SaO_2**	> 95%	< 95%	$S\bar{V}O_2$	60-80%	< 60%
SpO_2	> 95%	< 95%	$Ca-\bar{V}O_2$	4.5-5.0 mL/dL	↑↓
Efficiency					
$PA-aO_2$	10-25 mmHg (air) 30-50 mmHg (100%)	>25 mmHg	$O_{2_{ER}}$	25%	↑↓
			$\dot{V}O_2$	200-250 mL/min	↑↓
			$\dot{D}O_2$	750 - 1000 mL/min	↑↓
PaO_2/PAO_2	0.8-0.9	<0.6	VQI	0.8	↑↓
PaO_2/FIO_2	>300	<300			
$PA-aO_2/PaO_2$	<1.0	>1.0			
Qs/Q_T phys	2-5%	> 20%			

*Normal Variations: Due to age, FIO_2, or barometric pressure

Age: $PaO_2 \approx 110 - 1/2$ patient's age

**SaO_2 = calculated O_2 saturation from PaO_2

SpO_2 = Peripheral O_2 saturation - measured value of Hgb

Types of Hypoxemia, by Abnormal Values

Types		PAO_2	PaO_2	$PA\text{-}aO_2$	$Pa\text{-}vO_2$	$PaCO_2$	$PACO_2$	$Pa\text{-}ACO_2$
Atmospheric		↓	↓	N	N	↓	↓	N
Tidal		↓	↓	N ↑	N	↑	↑	N
Alveolar	Deadspace	N ↓	N ↓	N ↕	N ↕	N ↕	↓	↑
Alveolar	Absolute Shunt	N ↑	↓	↑	N	N ↕	N ↕	N ↕
Alveolar	V/Q Mismatch (relative shunt)	N	↓	↑	N	N ↕	N ↕	N ↕
Alveolar	Diffusion defect	N	N ↓	↑	N	N ↓	N ↓	N
Hemoglobic		N	N	N	N	N ↓	N ↓	N
Stagnant		N	↓	↑	↑↑	N ↕	N ↕	N ↕
Histotoxic		N	N	N	↓	N	N	N
Demand		*Any of the above*						

For details on values, see Equation Chapter

Hypoxemia
Levels of Hypoxemia

	PaO$_2$	SpO$_2$ %	(PaO$_2$) Clinical Notes
Mild Hypoxemia	60-79 mmHg	90-94%	
Moderate Hypoxemia	40-59 mmHg	75-89%	
Severe Hypoxemia	< 40 mmHg	< 75%	PaO$_2$ 30: loss of consciousness PaO$_2$ 20: anoxia- brain injury likely

Refractory Hypoxemia: Hypoxemia that shows no or little ↑ PaO$_2$ with ↑ FIO$_2$. -- Defined as < 5 mmHg ↑ PaO$_2$ with 0.1 ↑ FIO$_2$.
Responsive Hypoxemia: Hypoxemia that shows a significant ↑ PaO$_2$ with ↑ FIO$_2$. Defined as > 5 mmHg ↑ PaO$_2$ with 0.1 ↑FIO$_2$.

Hypoxemic Respiratory Failure
Known as: Type I Acute Respiratory Failure (ARF), Lung Failure, Oxygenation Failure, or Respiratory Insufficiency
Definition: The failure of the lungs and heart to provide adequate O$_2$ to meet metabolic needs.
Criteria: PaO$_2$ < 60 mmHg on FIO$_2$ ≥ 0.50 -or-
PaO$_2$ < 40 mmHg on any FIO$_2$ -and/or-
SaO$_2$ < 90 %

Signs & Symptoms of Acute Hypoxemia/Hypoxia (Relative order of appearance)		Signs & Symptoms of Chronic Hypoxemia/Hypoxia
Tachypnea	Confusion	Arrhythmias
Dyspnea	Euphoria	↓ CO
Pallor	Bradycardia	Clubbing (sometimes)
Tachycardia	Hypotension	Dyspnea
Hypertension	Nausea/vomiting	Irritability
Headache	Loss of coordination	Tiredness
Anxiety	Lethargy/weakness	Papilledema
Cyanosis	Tremors	Polycythemia
Arrhythmias	Hyper-active	Impaired judgment
Blurred or tunnel	reflexes	Myoclonic jerking
vision	Stupor	Pulmonary hyperten-
Impaired judgment	Coma ≈ 30 mm Hg	sion
	Death	

Types & Causes of Hypoxemia/Hypoxia

Types	Causes	Examples
Atmospheric	Insufficient O_2 available	$\downarrow$ FIO_2 : Drowning (no FIO_2); O_2 therapy error ($\downarrow$ FIO_2 < 0.21) $\downarrow$ PAO_2 : High altitude (PAO_2 $\downarrow$ 4 mmHg/1000 ft)
Tidal	**Hypoventilation** ($\uparrow$ $PaCO_2$ $\rightarrow$ $\downarrow$ PaO_2)	Many causes of pulmonary compromise
Alveolar	**1. Deadspace (alveolar)** (wasted ventilation; ventilation without perfusion) (V/Q)	**$\uparrow$ Alveolar deadspace :** a) Complete block: Pulmonary embolus (air, blood, fat, tumor) b) $\downarrow$ blood flow: Shock, cardiac arrest, $\uparrow$ PVR c) $\uparrow$V/$\downarrow$Q: $\uparrow$ MV and/or PEEP ($\uparrow$ lung zones 1+2 from $\uparrow$ Palv)
	2. Shunt **A) Absolute (True) Shunt** (Perfusion without ventilation; 0/Q) **B) Relative shunt** (perfusion with $\downarrow$ventilation; $\downarrow$V/Q) (V/Q mismatch, shunt effect, or venous admixture)	**Anatomical shunts:** Pleural, bronchial, thebesian veins, anatomical defects **Capillary shunts +/or Shunt effect:** a) Alveoli collapsed, fluid filled or blocked (complete or partial): ARDS, atelectasis (most common), cystic fibrosis, pneumonia, pneumothorax, pulmonary edema b) $\downarrow$ or no alveolar ventilation: Airway obstruction, asthma, COPD, position changes, secretions, etc.
	3. Diffusion Defect ($\uparrow$ a-c membrane thickness)	Fibrosis, Proteinosis, Sarcoidosis

Types	Causes	Examples
Hemoglobic	Blood abnormality ($\downarrow$ CaO_2)	Anemia, hemorrhage, sickle cell, CO poison Shift of oxyhemoglobin dissociation curve to right
Stagnant	Blood perfusion abnormality ($\downarrow$ O_2 transport)	CV failure, arrythmias, hemorrhage, shock
Histotoxic	Tissue can't metabolize O_2	Cyanide poisoning
Demand	$\uparrow$ Metabolic demand for more O_2 (which then causes one or more of the above hypoxemic conditions)	Burns, exercise, fever, hyperthyroidism

See Oakes' ABG Pocket Guide: Interpretation and Management for:
- Disinguishing between types of Hypoxemia
- Hypoxemia Diagnostic Algorithm
- Estimating Degree of Pulmonary Dysfunction

ABG Pocket Guide

10-83

Hypoxemia Diagnostic Algorithm

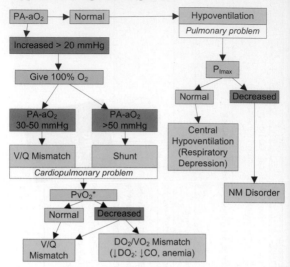

CO = Cardiac Output
* PvO_2 is obtained from a CVP line or PA catheter

Targets for Improving (Correcting) Oxygenation *

	PaO$_2$ (Goal)	SaO$_2$/SpO$_2$ (Goal)
Normal lung	≥80 mmHg	≥95%
Mild lung injury	≥70 mmHg	≥93%
Moderate lung injury	≥60 mmHg	≥90%
Severe lung injury **	≥55 mmHg	≥88%

*   Permissive hypoxemia is gaining interest/acceptance when there is concern for O$_2$ toxicity and/or VILI.

**   In shunts with > 50% FIO$_2$, ↑ FIO$_2$ has little to no effect. Therefore, in these situations (eg., ARDS) FIO$_2$ can be lowered to < 50% O$_2$ to reduce O$_2$ toxicity to the lungs without compromising PaO$_2$.

> **See Oakes' ABG Pocket Guide: Interpretation and Management of Oxygenation for:**
> • Evaluating Oxygenation Status
> • Lung Adequacy and Efficiency
> • Estimating Degree of Pulm. Dysfunction
> • Distinguishing Shunts, Deadspace, and Diffusion Defects
> • Assessment of Tissue Oxygen.
> • Management of Oxygenation
> • O2 Therapy for Vented Patients
> • (And More!)

See Equation Chapter for a Complete List of Oxygenation Equations

Oxygen Therapy for Adults in the Acute Care Facility[1]
(AARC CPG)

Indications

Acute MI

Hypoxemia (actual or suspected)

$PaO_2 < 60$ mm Hg

$SaO_2 < 90\%$

(or below desired) in adults, children, infants > 28 days in room air.

Severe trauma

Short-term therapy or postop

Precautions/Complications

Ventilatory depression: patients on an O_2 drive with elevated $PaCO_2$ and $PaO_2 \geq 60$ mm Hg.

$FIO_2 > 0.5$: absorption atelectasis, ↓ciliary function, ↓leukocyte function, fire hazard, bacterial contamination (humidification system), caution in patients with paraquat poisoning or receiving bleomycin, O_2 toxicity.

Contraindications

Monitoring

Patient:

Clinical assessment (pulm, CV, neuro status)

PaO_2 and/or SaO_2:

Upon initiation of therapy or within –

2 hours (COPD)

8 hours ($FIO_2 > 0.4$)

12 hours ($FIO_2 < 0.4$)

72 hours (acute MI)

Equipment:

q day or more frequent when: $FIO_2 > 0.5$, clinically unstable, heated gas mixture, artificial airway, blending systems.

Frequency

Continuous or intermittent (exercise, sleep)

1) Adapted from the AARC Clinical Practice Guidelines: Oxygen Therapy for Adults in the Acute Care Facility, 2002 Revision & Update *Respiratory Care*, Volume 47, #6, 2002.

OXYGEN DELIVERY DEVICES

Delivery System	Liter flow[1]	O₂% delivered[1]	Comments	Cautions
Low Flow System (Delivers 100% O₂ at flows < patient's inspiratory (demand). Room air is entrained, total patient demand is not met, and FIO₂'s highly variable.)				
Nasal Cannula	1-6 L/min	24-40%	Delivers approximately 4%/L, comfortable, good for low %, inexpensive, patient can eat, talk, and sleep.	$\downarrow$ FIO₂ as $\dot{V}_E$ $\uparrow$, need patent nasal passages, use humidifier ≥ 4 L/min, easily dislodged, may cause irritation, dryness, or nosebleed.
Nasal Catheter	1-6 L/min	24-45%	Same as cannula	Same as cannula, plus must be changed every 8 hours, clogs easily, abdominal distention.
Simple Mask	5-10 L/min	35-50%	Delivers approx. 4%/L, FIO₂ variable depending on fit and ventilation variables, hot/uncomfortable, interferes with eating/talking.	Need minimum 5 L/min to flush CO₂ from mask, more skin irritation
Partial Rebreathing Mask	6-10 L/min	40-70%	High % delivered, same as simple mask, FIO₂ variable depending on fit	$\dot{V}$ should be set to keep reservoir > 1/3 – 1/2 full upon inspiration.
Non-Rebreathing Mask	≥ 10 L/min	60-80%	Same as partial rebreathing mask	Same as partial rebreathing mask.

Delivery System	Liter flow[1]	O₂% delivered[1]	Comments	Cautions
High Flow System (High air flow with oxygen enrichment [HAFOE] which may meet the total demand of the patient [should be ≥ 60 L/min])				
Air Entrainment Mask (Venturi) **AIR ENTRAINMENT RATIOS**	Variable	24-50%	Exact O₂ concentrations, can be adapted to deliver aerosol, device of choice for patients on O₂ drive. O₂% — Air/O₂ ratio 24% — 25/1 28% — 10/1 30% — 8/1 35% — 5/1 40% — 3/1	Entrainment ports easily occluded. O₂% — Air/O₂ ratio 50% — 1.7/1 60% — 1/1 70% — 0.6/1 80% — 0.3/1
Calculating Oxygen Blending Ratios & Entrainment Ratios – See Equations, Chapter 9				
Air Entrainment Nebulizer or High-Volume Humidifier	8-40 L/min	28-100%	Used to deliver precise O₂ and/or aerosol, high O₂%, can provide controlled temperature of gas. FIO_2 determined by the nebulization system and flow rate or blender.	Use with aerosol mask, face tent, T-piece, trach mask or collar. May need two or three setups to meet inspiratory flow when FIO_2 > 50% Hazards of aerosol: (See aerosol therapy), condensation in tubing

10-88

Delivery System	Liter flow[1]	O₂% delivered[1]	Comments	Cautions
High-flow Therapy Systems	Neonatal: 1- 8 L/min Pediatric: 8-20 L/min Adult: 23-60 L/min	21% - 100% 30-100% (variable, dependent on pt flow requirement versus flow delivered)	Used to deliver precise O₂ and humidification from 80% to 100% RH at body temp (37º C). FIO₂ is determined by analysis via bleed-in or blender. Beneficial in adults with COPD, pulmonary fibrosis, CHF, asthma, CF and post-surgical care where low-flow oxygen or other delivery systems is inadequate Can also be used in humidifying CPAP, improving pulmonary hygiene, tracheostomy management and in the treatment of rhinitis/sinusitis.	Use with a special large-bore nasal cannula to accommodate high liter flows. Recommended for neo/ped pts with oxygenation difficulties related to BPD, CF and other pulm conditions w/ PaO₂ < 55 mmHg or SpO2 < 88%, tachypnea, retractions, mild apnea and/or bradycardia (AOP). Use in conjunction with SpO2 monitoring May create variable CPAP effect (some estimate as much as 1 cmH2O per 10 L/min, though may vary widely by device, physiology, etc.)

1) Based upon AARC Clinical Practice Guideline, Oxygen Therapy for Adults in the Acute Care Facility — 2002 Revision & Update, *Respiratory Care*, Vol 47, # 6, 2002.

Oxygen Conserving Devices (OCD)

OCDs provide oxygen on inspiration only, thereby reducing the amount of oxygen used. Due to individual patient variations, prescribed flows must be individually determined by SaO2 during rest and exercise.

Types of OCDs

Type	Advantages	Disadvantages
Reservoir Cannula "Mustache" or pendant	Least expensive to operate Reduces the amount of oxygen use	Conspicuous Expensive to buy and frequent replacement Heavy/cumbersome Uncomfortable
Pulse-dose or Demand-flow Systems (May be rate responsive)	Reduces the amount of oxygen use Some units switch to continuous flow if inspiration is not detected See * below	Annoying clicking noise If battery-powered, device must be maintained and recharged Cannot be used with oxygen concentrator Catheters and sensors may malfunction Cumbersome Nasal breathing required to trigger (perform nocturnal SpO2)

Continued on Next Page

Type	Advantages	Disadvantages
Transtracheal Oxygen System (TTOS) **	Improved compliance	Catheter dislodgment or lost tract
	Increased mobility	High cost
	Less accidental disruption during sleep; improved sleep	Humidification required
		Invasive procedure with complications: infection, bleeding, bronchospasm, and subQ emphysema
	Less facial/nasal/ear irritation (vs cannula)	
	May combine with a pulse-dosed oxygen device (oxygen use reduced even more)	Mucus plugging – requires daily cleaning, saline instillation, and maintenance and periodic replacement
	More cosmetically appealing	Not for all patients
	Reduces the amount of oxygen use	Requires significant self-care and patient education
	Senses of taste and smell are not affected	

!

It is not possible to calculate cylinder duration times when OCDs are in use because of 3 variables: cylinder size, setting on OCD regulator, and patient's actual respiratory rate. Most OCDs provide a savings ratio (i.e., 3:1, 4:1), which estimates the improved cylinder duration when compared to the continuous flow setting and helps better predict cylinder duration.

* Pulse-dose systems provide a bolus of O2 at a relatively high flow rate during only the first part of inspiration; demand-flow systems provide oxygen at the set flow throughout the inspiratory phase. Hybrid systems incorporate the features of pulse-dose and demand-flow (a large bolus of oxygen during the initial inspiratory phase followed by oxygen flow throughout the rest of inspiration).

** Indications for TTOS – Problems with standard devices: complications, cosmetics, inadequate oxygenation, need for improved mobility, poor compliance.

Relative contraindications of TTOS – Cardiac arrhythmias, compromised immune system, copious sputum, excessive anxiety, prolonged bleeding times, severe bronchospasm, uncompensated respiratory acidosis.

Heliox Therapy (Helium - Oxygen)	
Function	Helium reduces the resistance of air/O_2 flowing through narrowed airways. Its primary value is in the tx of airway obstruction by enhancing the delivery of O_2 and aerosol to the distal areas of the lung. Helium can be used as a temporizing agent to reduce WOB and allow time for the more standard forms of therapy to reach peak effect.
Indications	• Acute exacerbations of COPD or asthma • Post extubation stridor • Status asthmaticus • Tracheal stenosis • Upper airway obstruction

Benefits	• Improved homogeneity of gas distribution resulting in:
	  • ↑ alveolar ventilation, oxygenation and V_T,
	  • ↓ WOB, $PaCO_2$, gas trapping, auto-PEEP, PIP and Pplat, barotrauma, I:E ratios, and shunting
	• Movement of the equal-pressure point of the airways upstream

Common Mixtures	• 80% He / 20% O_2 • 70% He / 30% O_2 * (* Used when O_2 therapy is indicated for hypoxemia. If FIO_2 > 0.6 is required, He/O_2 will have little effect)

Administration	**Spontaneous breathing**: Deliver via tight-fit NRB. May add O_2 nasal cannula to titrate to desired SpO_2.
	
	Intubated: Deliver as adjunct via ventilator
	
	Delivery using an O_2 flowmeter requires flow conversion:
	  70/30: set flow x 1.6 = total flow delivered
	  80/20: set flow x 1.8 = total flow delivered

Monitoring	ABG sampling Arrhythmia Dyspnea (WOB & SOB)	Heart rate Pulse oximetry Pulsus paradoxus
Hazards	Anoxia- analyze delivered gas Barotrauma- via ventilators not designed for heliox	Too ↑ or too ↓ bronchodilator - too ↓ or ↑ of a flow through the neb Hypothermia - via hood on infants

11 DISEASES and DISORDERS

Continued Next Page

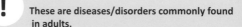

! These are diseases/disorders commonly found in adults.

- See **Oakes' Neonatal/Pediatric Respiratory Care** for neonatal and pediatric diseases/disorders.
- See **Oakes' Ventilator Management** for ventilation strategies for many of these diseases/disorders.
- See **RespiratoryUpdate.com** for Evidence-Based Guidelines and Expanded Disease Information.

Explanation of Key Used throughout this Chapter

	NAME - MOST COMMONLY ACCEPTED MEDICAL TERM LISTED IN ALPHABETICAL ORDER (OTHER NAMES OR ABBREVIATIONS)
Def	Definition
Types	When present, contains information regarding various types of disease or disorder
Etiology	**Origin** of disease or disease-causing organisms.
CM	**Clinical Manifestations** Listings indicate the most commonly found pulmonary manifestations (not all-inclusive). Manifestations of other body systems are generally not included.
CXR	**Chest X-Ray** - common findings
EBG	**Evidence-Based Guidelines** Available for Topic (Guidelines can be researched independently, or find direct links to information on RespiratoryUpdate.com)
CC	**Critical Care Considerations** - note that this will indicate material available in other Oakes' Pocket Guides, as well as online at RespiratoryUpdate.com.
Tx	**Treatment** Overview, including relevant algorithms based on latest Evidence-Based Medicine

Not every category will be presented for every disease - only those that have been deemed clinically relevant.

ACQUIRED IMMUNE DEFICIENCY SYNDROME (AIDS)

Definition	Infection with human immunodeficiency virus (HIV) which attacks CD4 T-lymphocytes of the immune system to produce a profound **immunosuppressed** state resulting in **opportunistic infections** and Kaposi's sarcoma.
Etiology	HIV, plus secondary infections of Pneumocystis, viral, bacterial, or mycoplasma pneumonia, and any other opportunistic infection. High Risk populations include multiple sexual partners, IV drug users, Hemophilia. **Stages:** 1. Viral Transmission 2. Acute HIV Infection 3. Seroconversion (4-10 weeks after viral transmission) 4. Clinical Latent Period (asymptomatic besides possible lymphadenopathy) 5. Early Symptomatic HIV Infection (P. Carinii in up to 50% of cases, bacterial PNA also possible) 6. AIDS (CD4 < 200 mm3 - symptomatic or asymptomatic) 7. Advanced HIV Infection (CD4 < 50 mm3) - 12-18 mos survival usually at this time
CM	Variable depending on cause of infection. Usually ↓ WBC, lymphocytes, and CD4 T cells (the lower the cell count, the greater the severity of infection).
CXR	Variable depending on type of infection. Note that CXR may be normal in pts with HIV who have no active secondary infection.
Tx	**Primary:** Antiretroviral Therapies Goals center around treating HIV viruses (HARRT) and aggressively addressing secondary infections. Current trends favor identifying specific causes of infection and treating those (versus empiric therapies).

ACTINOMYCOSIS	
Def	Chronic suppurative and granulomatous fungal infection which may cause pneumonia. It presents in three anatomic forms (1) cervicofacial, (2) thoracic, and (3) abdominal.
Etiology	*Actinomyces israelli* (not a true fungus) Gram+ rod, anaerobic. **Route**: aspiration or hemotogenous from an infected oral focus. May be normal oral flora, especially with decayed teeth. **Predisposing Conditions:** • Tooth Extractions or Eruptions • Gingivitis • Diabetes • Malnutrition • Immunosupression
CM	Disease manifests as pneumonia, which can be complicated by abscesses, empyema, and pleurodermal sinuses. Cough with purulent sputum, hemoptysis, empyema, chest pain on breathing, clubbing, constitutional symptoms.
CXR	Nonsegmental consolidation, cavitation.
Tx	Antibiotics (high-dose penicillin)

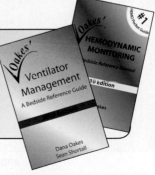

See Oakes' Ventilator Management and Oakes' Hemodynamic Monitoring for Critical Care Considerations for all relevant Diseases and Disorders

ACUTE RESPIRATORY DISTRESS SYNDROME (ARDS) AND ACUTE LUNG INJURY (ALI)

Def

An acute restrictive disease of diminishing FRC and severe hypoxia caused by injury to the alveolar – capillary membrane resulting in alveolar transudates, and ↓ surfactant, atelectasis, intrapulmonary shunting, ↑$\dot{V}D$, ↓ compliance and often multiple organ failure.

Definition according to the American-European Consensus Conference on ARDS, 1994:

1. **Acute onset of Respiratory Distress**

2. **Hypoxemia**:
   ARDS: P/F ratio < 200
   ALI: P/F ratio < 300

3. **Bilateral Consolidation on CXR**

4. **Absence of clinical finding of Cardiogenic Pulmonary Edema** (PAOP < 18 mmHg, or no LA HTN)

Etiology

Respiratory (Direct)	Non-Respiratory (Indirect)
• Aspiration	• Blood transfusion reactions
• Near-drowning	• Burns (massive)
• O₂ toxicity	• DIC
• Pneumonia (all types)	• Drug abuse
• Post-pneumonectomy	• Fat embolism
• Raised ICP (head injury)	• Pancreatitis (acute)
• Smoke inhalation	• Prolonged cardiopulmonary bypass
• Thoracic irradiation	• Sepsis
• Trauma (lung contusion/injury)	• Shock (severe, prolonged)
• Vasculitis	

ARDS - Continued Next Page

CM	**General**	• Agitated, anxious, confused, restless • Rapid-onset (hours- to days- post-insult)
	Respiratory	• Inspection (cough, cyanosis, dyspnea, retractions, tachypnea, ↑ WOB) • Palpation (↓ chest expansion) • Percussion (dull) • Auscultation (↓ BS, bronchial BS over consolidation, crackles)
	Pulm. Dyn	• ↓ C_L (total C < 30 mL/cm H_2O) • ↑PIP (vent) • ↓TC; ↑$\dot{V}_D$
	PFT's	• Restrictive pattern (↓ FRC)
	ABG's	• Oxygenation – refractory hypoxemia (PaO_2/FIO_2 ≤300), ↑ shunt (> 20%) • Ventilation – respiratory alkalosis → respiratory acidosis
	Cardiovasc.	• ↑ HR • PCWP < 15-18 mm Hg* • PAD – PCWP > 5mmHg
	Compare with CHF: PCWP > 15-18 mm Hg. (See also Pg 8-12)	
CXR	2-24 hrs: Diffuse alveolar and interstitial infiltrates (peripheral and dependent zones), air bronchograms.* 24-48 hrs: coalesce to produce massive air space consolidation in both lungs. * Compare with CHF: cardiomegaly, perihilar infiltrates, pleural effusion.	
EBG	• The American-European Consensus Conference on ARDS • Cochrane Reviews	
CC	• See **Oakes' Ventilator Management** for detailed Mechanical Ventilation Strategies • See **Oakes' Hemodyanmic Monitoring** for detailed Cardio-pulmonary Information	

ARDS - Continued Next Page

General Considerations:

- Treat underlying cause while providing needed Supports
- Maintain adequate oxygenation and ventilation: use Lung Protective strategies (see Oakes' Ventilator Management for detailed strategies)
- Use PEEP/CPAP to ↑FRC (lung recruitment maneuvers)
- Focus on Airway Clearance Therapies, Lung Expansion (see appropriate sections in Chapter 10 for further information)
- Diuretics as indicated
- Keep Oxygen consumption minimal
- Maintain hemodynamic stability and tissue perfusion

During progression of this inflammatory process, other strategies may be considered. Each one should be considered in light of evidence-based medicine, as well as risks-benefits:

- High-Frequency Ventilation (Oscillator)
- iNO Therapy
- Prone positioning
- ECMO
- Steroids
- Surfactant Therapy
- Inverse Ratio Modes of Ventilation (APRV)
- Antibiotics
- Permissive Hypercapnia (lung protection)

Tx

ALVEOLAR HYPOVENTILATION SYNDROMES

Def	Acute or chronic breathing disorder featuring inadequate alveolar ventilation, causing an increased $PaCO_2$.	

Etiology	Chest Wall Deformities	Kyphoscoliosis, etc.
	COPD	when FEV1 < 1.0 L or < 35% predicted
	Neuromuscular Disorders	Guillain-Barre Syndrome*, Myasthenia Gravis*, Muscular Dystrophy, ALS
	Obesity Hypoventilation Syndrome	Pickwickian. Gross obesity, may occur with OSA, decreased chemical drive to breathe, Lung wall restriction caused by weight on chest
	Primary (Central) Alveolar Hypoventilation	Central Respiratory Drive impairment (Ondine's Curse)

CM	*See Specific Diseases for Clinical Manifestations	
	Central Alveolar Hypoventilation:	SaO_2 decreases during sleep because of depressed ventilatory response to hypoxia and hypercapnia.
	Obesity Hypoventilation Syndrome	• Morbid Obesity • Hypoventilation • Hypersomnolence • Fragmented sleep • Hypercapnia, Hypoxemia • Acidemia (may be compensated) • Polycythemia • Cor Pulmonale • Systemic HTN during sleep

Tx	*See Specific Diseases for Treatment Strategies	
	Obesity Hypoventilation Syndrome	• Treat OSA (NPPV) • Encourage weight loss • Use PEEP/CPAP to offset chest wall • Recognize and Tx comorbidities • Consider trach in difficult-to-tx

	ALVEOLAR PROTEINOSIS (PAP) *(SEE ALSO INTERSTITIAL LUNG DISEASE)*
Def	Chronic, diffuse, progressive alveolar and interstitial deposition of phospholipoprotein derived from pulmonary surfactant. Links have been made with impaired macrophage maturation/function

Etiology	Two Forms:
	1. Primary (Idiopathic)
	2. Secondary
	  • Lung Infections
	  • Hematologic malignancies
	  • Inhalation of dusts (silica, aluminum, insecticides, etc.)
	  • Immune Dysfunction (AIDS, Niemann-Pick, etc.)
	
	Usuually occurs in people 20-50 years, though rarely may be present at birth

CM	Asymptomatic to death: • Persistent Cough – mild, nonproductive (or scant) • Progressive DOE • Fine Crackles • Hypoxemia (incl. clubbing) • Fatigue, Malaise • Pleuritic Chest Pain • Constitutional symptoms (affect many diff systems) • Samples via BAL appear milky Mortality Rates generally < 10 %
CXR	Diffuse, bilateral, feathery, butterfly or "bat's wing" pattern.
Tx	• If asymptomatic or minimally symptomatic, may consider observation with no interventions • Bronchial hygiene and lung lavage with normal saline if a-A gradient > 40 mmHg; Dyspnea/Hypoxemia at rest or on exertion; PaO2 < 65 mmHg on RA • Consideration for Blood Stimulating Factor Treatments • If persistent, consideration for lung transplantation

ASPERGILLOSIS	
Def	Variety of fungal infections marked by an inflammatory granulomatous lesions and aspergillomas (fungus balls). Usually superimposed on individuals with underlying immunosuppression.
Types	**Allergic bronchopulmonary aspergillosis** (ABPA) – asthmatics allergic to Aspergillosis antigen, may present with eosinophilia. **Fungal ball aspergillosis** – fungal ball in cavities. **Invasive aspergillosis** (rare) – chronic necrotizing pneumonia with abscess formation.
Etiology	*Aspergillus fumigatus/niger* (most common). Spores found in soil, decaying organic matter, or building materials. Maybe normal flora in mouth or sputum. **Route** – inhalation or GI tract.
CM	**Asymptomatic to death** – cough with minimal mucoid sputum, recurrent hemoptysis, fever, recurrent pulmonary infections.
CXR	Highly variable – nodules, lesions, nonsegmental consolidation, abscess formation, fungal balls, air cavities, dilated bronchi.
EBG	• Clinical Practice Guidelines of the Infectious Diseases Society of America: Treatment of Aspergillosis
Tx	Depends on type – ranges from bronchial hygiene and anti-fungals to resection. ABPA - oral corticosteroids, azole anti-fungal

ASPIRATION PNEUMONIA / PNEUMONITIS

Def	**Aspiration pneumonia**: lung infection caused by chronic aspiration of colonized oropharyngeal secretions. **Aspiration pneumonitis**: acute lung inflammation following aspiration of gastric contents.
Etiology	Aspiration of bacteria from oropharynx, GI tract, or ventilator circuit condensate. VAP = ventilator associated pneumonia Aspiration of food particles and acid (↑severity as pH↓) **Contributing Factors:** • Anesthesia/alcohol/drugs • Convulsions, CPR • Depressed mental function • Inadequate cough mechanism • Impaired gastric emptying • Impairment of swallowing mechanism

CM	**Pneumonia (PNA)**	Signs of infection with purulent sputum
	Pneumonitis	Sudden tachypnea and dyspnea, cough, crackles, wheezing, cyanosis, hypoxemia, may progress to respiratory failure. PFTs variable

CXR	Patchy, mottled, segmental consolidation (depending on position when aspirated), atelectasis, abscess.
Tx	• Preventive Measures • Airway Clearance (suction) • Oxygen Therapy • Bronchodilators • Therapeutic Bronchoscopy • Invasive ventilatory support, if severe • Antibiotics if indicated • Steroids

	ASTHMA	
Def	A chronic inflammatory disorder of the airways. Airway hyperresponsive, resulting in reversible or partially reversible airway obstruction, that leads to recurrent episodes of wheezing, breathlessness, chest tightness, and coughing.	
Types	**Extrinsic** (allergic) asthma: 90% of all asthma; typically develops in childhood	
	Intrinsic (non-allergic) asthma: 10% of all asthma; develops after age of 30 to 40	

Etiology	**Inhalation**	• Genetic?
		 • **Allergens:**
		   • Animal (dander, urine, etc)
		   • Cockroach feces
		   • House dust mites
		   • Indoor fungi (mold)
		   • Outdoor (pollen, spores)
		 • **Occupational exposure:**
		   • Dust, gases, fumes, chemicals
		 • **Irritants:** Air pollution, odors, sprays, stove fumes, tobacco smoke

	Other Factors	• Cold air, exercise • Drugs, food • Emotional stress • Gastroesophageal reflux • Rhinitis/sinusitis • Sensitivity to drugs (aspirin, beta-blockers, nonsteroidal anti-inflammatory, sulfites) • Viral respiratory infections

CM	Agitation/restless Anxiety Chest tightness Cough Diaphoresis Dyspnea/SOB Flaring	↑RR, ↑HR ↑TE, ↑WOB Hyperinflation Hyperresonance Hypoxemia Pulsus paradoxus Retractions	Wheezing* Late signs: ↓$PaCO_2$ (initial)* → ↑$PaCO_2$ (late) ↓ BS Cyanosis
	DANGER: Respiratory Distress without wheezing (silent chest), or ABG with normal $PaCO2$ (pt tiring) may indicate impending Respiratory Failure		

	Is it Asthma? *

CM (cont.)	*The presence of any of these signs and symptoms should increase the suspicion of asthma:*
	• Wheezing (but don't exclude consideration if not present)
	• History of:
	  - Cough, worse at night
	  - Recurrent wheeze, difficult breathing, or chest tightness
	• Symptoms occur or worsen at night, awakening the patient
	• Patient also has eczema, hayfever, or family hx of asthma
	• Symptoms occur or worsen in the presence of: (see etiology above)
	• Symptoms respond to anti-asthma therapy
	• Patient's colds "go to the chest" or take more than 10 days to clear
	
	* Adapted from Global Initiative for Asthma (GINA), 2007.
	
	PFTs: Obstructive Pattern
	↓FVC,↓FEV & FEV₁%,↓PEF ---- ↑FRC, ↑RV, ↑TLC

CXR	Hyperinflation, ↑bronchial markings, flat diaphragm, ↑rib spaces, more radiolucent, narrow heart shadow.

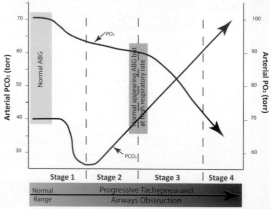

Arterial blood gas, ABG, during various stages of asthma.

11-14

<table>
<tr><td>EBG</td><td>

- American College of Chest Physicians - Inhaled Corticosteroid Use in Asthma
- American Thoracic Society/European Respiratory Society Statement: Asthma Control and Exacerbations
- Cochrane Reviews
- NHLBI Guidelines for the Diagnosis and Treatment of Asthma (Expert Panel Report 3)
- Global Strategy for Asthma Management and Prevention - Global Initiative for Asthma (GINA)

</td></tr>
<tr><td>CC</td><td>See Oakes Ventilator Management for detailed Mechanical Ventilation strategies related to Asthma</td></tr>
</table>

Levels of Asthma Control*

Characteristic	Controlled (all of the following)	Partly controlled (any measure present in any week)	
Daytime symptoms	None (≤ 2/week)	> 2/week	
Limitations of Activities	None	Any	
Nocturnal symptoms/ awakening	None	Any	3+ features of partly controlled asthma present in any week
Need for reliever/rescue treatment	None (≤ 2/week)	> 2/week	
Lung Function (PEF or FEV$_1$)	Normal	< 80% pred or personal best	
Exacerbations	None	≥ 1 /year	1 in any week

* Adapted from Global Initiative for Asthma (GINA), 2007. See below.

11-15

Asthma Severity, Control, and Treatment

Classifying Severity of Asthma Exacerbations *

Parameter[1]	Mild	Moderate	Severe	Respiratory Arrest Imminent
Breathless	Walking, can lie down	Talking, prefers sitting	At rest, hunched forward	
Talks in	Sentences	Phrases	Words	
Alertness	May be agitated	Usually agitated	Usually agitated	Drowsy or confused
RR[2]	↑	↑	Often > 30/min	
Accessory Muscle Use	None	Usually	Usually	Paradoxical Breathing
Wheeze	Moderate, end-expir	Loud	Usually loud	Absent
Pulse[3]	<100	100-120	> 120	< 60
Pulsus paradoxus	Absent, < 10mmHg	May be present, 10-25 mmHg	Often present, > 25 mmHg[7]	Absent? = respiratory fatigue?
PEF[4]	> 80%	60-80%	< 60% [5]	
PaO2 (on RA)	Normal	> 60mmHg	< 60 mmHg	
PaCO2 [6]	< 45mmHg	< 45 mmHg	> 45 mmHg	
SaO2 (on RA)	> 95%	91-95%	< 90%	

1. The presence of several parameters, but not necessarily all, indicates the general classification of the attack.
2. Normal RR for children: < 2 mo, < 60/min; 2-12 mo, < 50/min; 1-5 yrs, < 40/min; 6-8 yrs, < 30/min.
3. Normal pulse for children: infants (2-12 mo), < 160/min; pre-school (1-2 yrs), < 120/min; school age (2-8 yrs), < 110/min.
4. After initial bronchodilator, % pred or % personal best.
5. < 100 L/min adults or response lasts < 2 hrs.
6. Hypercapnia develops more readily in young children than in adults and adolescents.
7. 20-40 mm Hg in children

	Treatment Strategies See Severity Chart (11-16) for details on Symptoms of Distress	
ASTHMA Tx (continued)	**General Therapy** **(Mild to Moderate Symptoms)**	• Oxygen Therapy should be given to all pts in respiratory distress • Follow oxygenation via SpO2 or A-Line • Maintain SpO2 > 90% • Aggressive hydration may be indicated for infants/small children, but is not recommend for older children • CPT, mucolytics and sedation are generally not recommended • Consider Steroids, Bronchodilators (scheduled and PRN)
	(Moderate to Severe Symptoms)	• Consider Albuterol via Continuous Nebulizer (10+ mg/hr) • Heliox if reasonable hypoxemia • I.V. Steroids
	Respiratory Failure	• Do not delay Intubation once it is indicated • Use of NPPV is controversial, but may support pt's ventilatory needs for a short trial • During BVM, be aware of high risk of air-trapping • May continue Steroids and high-dose bronchodilators when on MV support. • Aim for early extubation post-crisis
	Post-Crisis	• Utilize opportunity to do comprehensive education post-crisis. Discussion should include use of an Asthma Plan, Pt demonstration of proper use of medications, as well as indications, etc. • Include family supports as appropriate • Include environmental review (triggers) • Connect pt with Asthma Educator/Program when available. Bilingual services may be available. • Emphasize the controllable nature of Asthma.

ATELECTASIS	
Def	Incomplete expansion, non-aeration, and/or collapse of alveoli.
Etiology	**Absorption/Obstructive** - absorption of gas from the alveoli after bronchial obstruction (acute: mucous plug, spasm, foreign body; subacute: 100% O_2, retained secretions, tumor).
	Compression - compression of lung parenchyma by a space occupying lesion (tumor, pleural effusion, tension pneumothorax).
	Hypoventilation - low V_T (anesthesia, drugs, CNS disorder, fatigue, splinting, tight chest dressings, prolonged bed rest, MV)
	Micro/Miliary - widespread collapse of alveoli due to loss of or interference with surfactant (e.g., ARDS, O_2 toxicity).
	Passive - normal lung retraction when lung is separated from the chest wall (e.g., pneumothorax, pleural effusion).
	Post-op - ↓lung expansion (↓ cough and deep breathing)
CM	Asymtomatic to ↑ dyspnea / ↑ WOB ↑ RR / ↑ HR ↓ chest expansion Tracheal shift (same side)	Chest pain, fever, restless Refractory hypoxemia (capillary shunting) **PFTs** – restrictive	**Auscultation over affected area:** late crackles, ↓ BS if airway obstructed, bronchial BS if airway patent, ↑ fremitus, dull percussion note
CXR	Local opacification, air bronchograms, narrowing of rib spaces, elevation of diaphragm on affected side, displacement of heart and trachea towards affected side (unless compression). Micro type = diffuse reticular granular pattern
Tx	Correct underlying cause. Lung inflation therapy, O_2 therapy, bronchial hygiene, CPAP or MV.

BACTERIAL PNEUMONIAS

Def	Inflammation of the lungs resulting from a bacterial infection

Types

Atypical: Pneumonia caused by *Mycoplasma*, *Chlamydia* and/or *Legionella*

Bacteriodes species: Anerobic g-neg rods. Common with bronchiectasis.

Enterobacteria (*Pseudomonas aeruginosa*, *Escherichia coli*, *Proteus species*). Anerobic g-neg rods. Usually nosocomial, common with bronchiectasis, chronic bronchitis, cystic fibrosis.

Klebsiella pneumoniae: Anerobic g-neg rods. Similar to pneumococcus, plus necrotizing. Common in diabetic, alcoholic, and chronic lung disease patients.

Haemophilus influenza: Anaerobic, g-neg coccobacilli. Common in COPD.

Legionella pneumophila: Anaerobic, g-neg rod like. Found in contaminated water systems. Causes Legionnaire's disease.

Mycoplasma pneumoniae: viral like organism, community acquired from inhalation of droplet nuclei (use resp. isolation), most common cause of nonbacterial pneumonia (See viral pneumonia)

Serratia marscesens: Anaerobic, g-neg bacilli. May cause pseudohemoptysis, commonly grows in respiratory equipment.

Staphylococcus aureus: Aerobic g-pos cocci. Most common bronchopneumonia (use strict resp. isolation), necrotizing.

Streptococcus pneumoniae: Aerobic g-pos cocci (diplococci). Formerly called pneumococcal pneumonia, 2/3 of all bacterial pneumonia. Often follows URI.

Streptococcus pyogenes: Aerobic g-pos cocci. Usually follows URI, maybe necrotizing.

Etiology

Route: aspiration, inhalation, direct infection via blood.

Predisposing factors: alcoholism, cardiac failure, pre-existing lung disease (asthma, CF, COPD), ↓ cough, debilitation, ET tube, immobility, immuno-compromise, malnutrition, old age, recent smoking, viral respiratory infection.

CM	**May have Rapid Onset of Symptoms, which could be Fatal** • Chills/ Fever • Cough • Cyanosis • Dyspnea / ↑ WOB • Headache/Malaise • ↑RR, ↑HR • Pleural pain • Sputum (See Ch 5) • Tachypnea • Warm, flushed skin • Crackles/ wheeze • Pleural rub (possible) • Bronchial BS/dull percussion over consolidation
CXR	**Lobar** – homogeneous consolidation with well-defined margins. **Bronchial** – patchy, bilateral, peri-bronchial consolidation. **Both** – pleural effusion, cavitation.
EBG	• Infectious Diseases Society of America/American Thoracic Society Consensus Guidelines on the Management of Community-Acquired Pneumonia in Adults • Guidelines for the Management of Adults with Hospital-Acquired, Ventilatior-Associated, and Healthcare-Asso-ciated Pneumo nia, Official Statement of the American Thoracic Society and the Infectious Diseases Society of America.
Tx	• Antibiotics • Airway Clearance • O_2 therapy. • Pts with more significant infections/manifestations may require Mechanical Ventilation

BLASTOMYCOSIS	
Def	Fungal infection initially affecting the lungs, followed by hematogenous dissemination to other organs. Diagnosed via histology
Etiology	*Blastomyces dermatitidis*: inhabits soil, Southeast USA, Mississippi valley, along Great Lakes and St Lawrence river. **Route**: inhalation of spores. Higher Risk: Adults who hunt, fish, camp, operate equipment in high-risk geographical areas
CM	Most acutely infected patients are asymptomatic (or self-limited). Otherwise generally develops into a chronic pneumonia: • Persistent chest pain & tightness, • Dyspnea • Cough • Purulent (bloody or brown) sputum • Low-grade fever • Weight loss • Headache, fatigue, malaise. • May mimic bacterial pneumonia. • Severe cases may develop into ARDS and Resp Failure • Other Systems: • Skin: Lesions with purplish hue around them • Osteoarticular involvement • Prostatitis or epididymitis • Chronic Meningitis (rare)
CXR	Highly variable segmental or lobar consolidation with cavitation. May include pulmonary nodules (cavitating or non)
EBG	• Clinical Practice Guidelines for the Management of Blastomycosis, Infectious Diseases Society of America
Tx	• Systemic Anti-fungal drugs (azoles) • Amphotericin B for severe or life-threatening disease. Once controlled, change to azoles • Airway Clearance, and other Supportive Therapies, as Indicated

	BRONCHIECTASIS
Def	Abnormal, permanent dilatation and distortion of one or more conducting airways due to destruction of the elastic and muscular components of the bronchial wall.
Types	**Cylindrical**: Straight tube with abrupt widening **Saccular** (cystic): Outpouchings that balloon outward **Varicose** (fusiform): Gradual widening and tapering
Etiology	**Acquired bronchiectasis**: Necrosis due to frequent or long-standing airway blockage (inhaled foreign object, tumor, or mucus accumulation), infection, immune rx, or noxious chemicals. **Congenital bronchiectasis**: Abnormal airway development.
CM	Range; Asymptomatic - Death • Chronic cough – sputum volume varies, maybe mucopurulent, fetid sputum (settles into 3 layers: mucous, saliva, pus) • Hemoptysis / Recurrent infections • DOE • Crackles/wheezes • Clubbing • Hypoxemia leading to cor pulmonale • Weight loss
CXR	Normal to increased bronchovascular markings.
Tx	Prophylaxis, treat infections, control secretions, remove obstructions, treat complications (hemoptysis, hypoxemia, respiratory failure, cor pulmonale), resection?

CARBON MONOXIDE POISONING

Def

Inhalation of CO causing an inhibition of transport, delivery, and utilization of oxygen (decreased SaO_2 & CaO_2, left shift of O_2-Hgb curve, inhibits cytochrome c oxidase).

Etiology

Auto exhaust, home exhaust, space heaters, obstructed chimney, incomplete combustion of organic materials.

CM

Note: patients do not typically appear "cherry red" and PaO_2 and SpO_2 are usually normal!

Saturation of blood (COHb%)	Symptoms	FICO
0-10%	None	
10-20%	Tightness across forehead, slight headache, dilation of skin vessels.	0.007-0.012
20-30%	Headache, throbbing in temples	0.012-0.022
30-40%	Severe headache, weakness, dizziness, dimness of vision, nausea, vomiting, collapse, syncope, ↑HR, ↑RR.	0.022-0.035
40-50%	Above, plus ↑ tendency to collapse and syncope, ↑HR, ↑RR.	0.035-0.052
50-60%	↑HR, ↑RR, syncope, Cheyne-Stokes respiration, coma with intermittent convulsions.	0.052-0.080
60-70%	Coma with intermittent convulsions, depressed heart action and respiration, death possible.	0.080-0.120
70-80%	Weak pulse, depressed respiration, respiratory failure, death.	0.120-0.195

These are general guidelines. Some patients may be asymptomatic until COHb% > 40%

11-23

Clinical symptoms and COHb levels often do not coincide –
Treat whichever is the most severe.

> 10% COHb, w/ headache, or blurred vision:	Give 100% oxygen. Use tight fitting non-rebreather mask, ET tube, or other. Continue until < 10 %.
> 15% COHb:	100% O_2, plus admit to hospital if history of heart disease.
> 25% COHb abnormal neuro or CV exam, unconscious, severe acidosis, pregnant woman, or age > 60:	Give 100% O_2, plus transport to hyperbaric chamber is highly recommended.

Tx

Half-Life of COHb

In Air	300 minutes
In 100% O_2	90 minutes
@ 2.5 ATA (hyperbarics)	30 minutes

- Monitor Cardiac, ABG's and COhb level
- Intubate and ventilate if unconscious or uncooperative
- Avoid hyperventilation and $NaHCO_3$ (shifts oxy-heme curve to left)
- Steroids or hypothermia?
- Watch for latent deterioration (usually 4-9 days later), pulmonary edema, MI, CHF. Hyperbaric oxygenation (HBO) within 24 hrs of hospitalization reduces the risk for cognitive sequelae compared with standard normobaric O_2 therapy.

	CARDIAC TAMPONADE
Def	Acute, abnormal accumulation of fluid in pericardial sac resulting in heart compression.
Etiology	Hemorrhage (aneurysm, rupture, trauma) or pericarditis (infection, MI, surgery).
CM	Proportional to degree of heart compression (asymptomatic to total CV collapse), pulsus paradoxus, sinus tachycardia, Beck's triad (JVD [or ↓CVP], ↓BP, muffled heart).
CXR	Cardiac enlargement (water bottle shape), clear lungs
CC	See Oakes' Hemodynamic Monitoring for comprehensive information on Cardiac Tamponade
Tx	• Immediate pericardiocentesis • Maintain adequate CO • O_2 therapy as needed • Pericardiectomy?

	CHRONIC BRONCHITIS
Def	**Bronchitis** - inflammation of bronchial mucosa due to infection or chemical inhalation. **Chronic** - cough with excessive mucus production occurring on most days for at least three consecutive months for 2 years in a row. **Chronic bronchitis** – diagnosis based on symptomatology; a principal manifestation of COPD.
Etiology	Chronic irritation (smoking, air pollution), infections (viral, bacterial), hereditary.
CM	**See COPD** for Clinical Manifestations, CXR, Evidence-Based Guidelines, and Treatment Strategies

CHRONIC OBSTRUCTIVE PULMONARY DISEASE (COPD)

Def	A preventable and treatable disease with some significant extrapulmonary effects that may contribute to the severity in individual patients. Its pulmonary component is characterized by airflow limitation that is not fully reversible. The airflow limitation is usually progressive and associated with an abnormal inflammatory response of the lung to noxious particles or gases. *Asthma is not classified as COPD based on ATS Standards, 1995*
Etiology	*See Chronic Bronchitis and Emphysema* • The chronic airflow limitation characteristic of COPD is caused by a mixture of small airway disease (obstructive bronchiolitis) and parenchymal destruction (emphysema), the relative contributions of which vary from person to person. **Diagnosis:** • A diagnosis of COPD should be considered in any pt who has dyspnea (persistent and progressive), chronic cough, or sputum production and/or a history of exposure to risk factors, especially cigarette smoking, occupational dusts and chemicals, and/or indoor/outdoor pollution. • The diagnosis should be confirmed by spirometry (FEV_1, FVC, FEV_1/FVC ratio < 70%) • There may be a genetic component to COPD: Alpha-1 Antitrypsin Disorder (Alpha-1). The ATS, AARC, and ACCP all recommend routine, blood-based testing for Alpha-1 in all patients with suspected COPD. [1] • Research shows the greater the number of comorbidities, the more severe the Dyspnea in patients with COPD. [1]
EBG	• ACCP, ATS, ERS • GOLD • Cochrane Reviews • ICSI
CC	• See Oakes' Hemodynamic Monitoring for detailed Cardiopulmonary Function • See Oakes' Ventilator Management for detailed Mechanical Ventilation Strategies

Sandhaus, Robert A., MD, PhD, FCCP. AARC Professor Rounds, 2011, Management of the COPD Patient with Comorbidities

Comparison of Clinical Manifestations*

Characteristic	Emphysema (Pink Puffer)	Chronic Bronchitis (Blue Bloater)
Inspection		
Body	thin	stocky or fat (bloater)
Chest	barrel chest	normal
	hypertrophy of accessory muscles	↑ use of accessory muscles
Breathing Pattern	progressive dyspnea	variable
	labored (puffer)	normal
	retractions	normal
	↓ chest movement	normal
	↓ IE ratio, ↑ T_E	↑IE ratio, ↓ T_E
Posture	orthopnea	varibale
Cough	slight	considerable
Sputum	small amt - mucoid	large amt - purulent
Color	normal (pink)	cyanosis (blue)
Palpation	norm to ↓ fremitus	norm to ↓ fremitus
Auscultation		
BS	↓	norm to ↓
Wheezing	slight	episodic
Blood Gases		
PaO_2 resting	Slight ↓	Mod to Severe ↓
PaO_2 exercise	falls	stable
$PaCO_2$	norm	↑
HCO_3	norm	↑
PFT's**		
Spirometry	obstructive	obstructive
RV and TLC	↑	norm to ↓
Diffusion Capacity	↓	normal
Compliance	↑	normal
Hematocrit	< 55%	> 55%
ECG	right axis deviation	RVH
CXR		
Broncho-vascular markings	↓	↑
Hyperinflation	yes	no
Bullae/blebs	yes	no
Past History	normal	freq resp infections
Lifespan	norm (60-80 yrs)	shorter (40-60 yrs)
Cor pulmonale	uncommon	common
Death	nonpulmonary or RF	RVF or RF

See also Pg 1-16, 8-12 and Oakes' *Hemodynamic Monitoring: A Bedside Reference Manual* for greater detail.

* Pure chronic bronchitis or emphysema is rarely seen. Most commonly it is a combination of both.

** The diagnosis of COPD is confirmed by spirometry: the presence of a post-bronchodilator FEV_1 < 80% predicted, plus an FEV_1/FVC < 70%.

The following section is a brief summary of the Global Strategy for the Diagnosis, Management and Prevention of COPD, Global Initiative for Chronic Obstructive Lung Disease (GOLD) 2007. Available from: http://www.goldcopd.org.

Stages of COPD

Severity	Symptoms	Spirometry	Treatment
Stage I: Mild	Chronic cough and sputum (maybe)	FEV_1/FVC < 70% $FEV_1 \geq 80\%$ predicted	Avoid risk factors Obtain flu vaccine Short-acting bronchodilator prn
Stage II: Moderate	Progression of above, plus DOE	FEV_1/FVC < 70% FEV_1 50% to 79% predicted	Above, plus regular tx with one or more long-acting broncho- dilators and rehabilitation.
Stage III: Severe	↑ SOB and repeated exacerbations	FEV_1/FVC < 70% FEV_1 30% to 49% predicted	Above, plus inhaled gluco- corticosteroids if repeated exacerbations
Stage IV: Very Severe	Impaired quality of life and exacerbations maybe life threatening	FEV_1/FVC < 70% FEV_1 <30% pred or < 50%, plus chronic respiratory failure or RHF	Above, plus long-term oxygen therapy if chronic resp. failure. Consider surgical tx.

The Four Components of COPD Management
1) Assess and Monitor
2) Reduce Risk Factors
3) Manage Stable COPD
4) Manage Exacerbations

1) Assess and Monitor

- Detailed medical history
- ABG's (see below)
- Bronchodilator reversibility test
- CXR
- Spirometry
- Alpha-1 antitrypsin deficiency screen (family Hx or < 45 yrs)

2) Reduce Risk Factors

Smoking cessation, minimize occupational exposures and indoor/outdoor pollutions.

3) Managing Stable COPD

Do's:

ABGs should be considered for patients with FEV1 < 50 % predicted or signs of respiratory failure (central cyanosis, PaO_2 < 60 mm Hg +/or SaO_2 < 90% (room air) with or without $PaCO_2$ > 50 mm Hg) or RHF (ankle swelling and↑ JV pressure).

Bronchodilator drugs: (central to symptom management)
- β2-agonists, anticholinergics, and methylxanthines – choice depends on availability and patient's response.
- Inhaled therapy is preferred
- Long-acting inhaled are more effective and convenient.
- Combining bronchodilators may improve efficacy and ↓ side effects compared to ↑ dose of a single bronchodilator.
- Wet nebulizers may provide subjective benefit in acute episodes.
- In general, nebulized therapy for a stable patient is not appropriate unless shown to be better than conventional dose therapy.

Inhaled glucocorticosteroids may reduce the risk of repeated hospitalizations and death. They should be considered for patients with an $FEV_1 < 50\%$, repeated exacerbations requiring oral steroids, and/or objective evidence of response to a trial of inhaled corticosteroids.

O_2 therapy: Keep PaO_2 at least 60 mm Hg and/or SaO_2 at least 90% (at rest).

Long-term O_2 therapy (> 15 hrs/day) is generally introduced at Stage IV in patients with: 1) $PaO_2 \leq 55$ mm Hg or $SaO_2 \leq 88\%$ on room air, with or without hypercapnia.; or 2) PaO_2 55 - 60 mm Hg or $SaO_2 \leq 88\%$ on room air, if there is evidence of pulmonary hypertension, peripheral edema (CHF), or hematocrit > 55%.

Patient education: Smoking cessation (The 5 As –See Ch 12), etc.

Systemic steroids are clinically beneficial to patients hospitalized with an exacerbation. (Chronic therapy should be avoided).

Don'ts:

Antibiotics, other than for treating infectious exacerbations, are not recommended.

Antitussives: regular use is not recommended.

Mast cell stabilizers or leukotriene modifiers are not recommended.

Mucolytic agents are generally not recommended.

N-acetylcysteine (antioxidant) may or may not have a role in treating exacerbations.

Nitric oxide is contraindicated.

4) Managing Exacerbations

Diagnosis of an Exacerbation

↑ breathlessness, often accompanied by wheezing and chest tightness ↑ cough and purulent sputum (altered color +/or tenacity), and fever.	Also may present with ↑RR, ↑HR, malaise, insomnia, fatigue, depression, and confusion.

Note: The most important sign of severe exacerbation is a change in mental status!

Assessing Severity of an Exacerbation

ABGs:

- Respiratory failure = room air PaO_2 < 60 mm Hg, &/or SaO_2 < 90% with or without $PaCO_2$ > 50 mm Hg
- Mechanical ventilation is indicated when pH < 7.36, $PaCO_2$ > 45-60 mm Hg, and PaO_2 <60 mm Hg.

Chest x-ray: identify complications/alternative diagnoses mimicking an exacerbation.

ECG: helps identify RV hypertrophy, arhythmias, and ischemic episodes.

Note: Low BP and inability to ↑ PaO_2 may suggest pulmonary embolism

Spirometry: is not recommended

Management

Indications for ICU Admission:

- Severe unresponsive dyspnea, confusion, lethargy, coma
- Life threatening ABGs (severe or worsening PaO_2 < 40 mm Hg, and/or $PaCO_2$ > 60 mm Hg, and/or pH < 7.25, despite O_2 and NIPPV therapy)
- Invasive MV and/or
- Hemodynamic instability (vasopressors needed).

Bronchodilator therapy: Short-acting, inhaled B2-agonists are preferred. If prompt response does not occur, then anticholinergics recommended. Role of aminophylline is controversial.

Glucocorticosteroids: Oral or intravenous are recommended as an addition to bronchodilator therapy.

O2 Therapy: Maintain PaO_2 > 60 mm Hg, SaO_2 > 90%. Check 30 min after initiating O_2 therapy.

CPT and PD: May be beneficial if > 25 mL sputum/day or lobar atelectasis.

Antibiotics: Give –

- With ↑ dyspnea, sputum volume and/or purulence
- When MV is required

Respiratory stimulants (doxapram) are not recommended.

Ventilation: See Oakes' ***Ventilator Management: A Bedside Reference Guide*** for indications and a detailed discussion.

Management of Severe but Not Life-Threatening Exacerbations of COPD in the Emergency Department or the Hospital

- Assess severity of symptoms, ABGs, CXR
- Administer controlled O_2 therapy and repeat ABG after 30-60 min
- Bronchodilators:
    - Increase doses or frequency
    - Combine β2-agonists and anticholinergics
    - Use spacers or air-driven nebulizers
    - Add IV methylxanthine, if needed
- Add glucocorticosteroids — Oral or intravenous.
- Consider antibiotics with signs of bacterial infection
    - oral or occasionally intravenous
- Consider NPPV
- At all times:
    - Monitor fluid balance and nutrition
    - Consider subcutaneous heparin
    - Identify/treat associated conditions (e.g., heart failure, arrhythmias)
    - Closely monitor condition of the patient

See:

1. *Global Strategy for the Diagnosis, Management and Prevention of COPD*, 2007 Update, Global Initiative for Chronic Obstructive Lung Disease (GOLD). Available from: www.goldcopd.org.
2. **Standards for the Diagnosis and Treatment of Patients with COPD**: A Summary of the ATS/ERS Position Paper, 2004. Available from: www.thoracic.org.

Also, see Oakes' *Ventilator Management: A Bedside Reference Guide* for further details and strategies for mechanical ventilation of the COPD patient.

COPD MANAGEMENT ALGORITHM[1,2]
(Therapy at each Stage)

[1] 1- Postbronchodilator FEV$_1$ is recommended for the diagnosis and assessment of severity of COPD.

2- Adapted from the *Global Strategy for the Diagnosis, Management and Prevention of COPD*. Global Initiative for Chronic Obstructive Lung Disease (GOLD), 2006.

I: MILD	II: MODERATE	III: SEVERE	IV: VERY SEVERE
FEV$_1$/FVC < 0.70	FEV$_1$/FVC < 0.70	FEV$_1$/FVC < 0.70	FEV$_1$/FVC < 0.70
FEV$_1$ ≥ 80% predicted	50% ≤ FEV$_1$ < 80% predicted	30% ≤ FEV$_1$ < 50% predicted	FEV$_1$ < 30% predicted or FEV$_1$ <30% predicted + chronic respiratory failure

Active reduction of risk factor(s); influenza vaccination

ADD short-acting bronchodilator (when needed)

ADD regular treatment with one or more long-acting bronchodilators (when needed); Add rehabilitation

ADD inhaled glucocorticosteroids if repeated exacerbations

ADD long-term O$_2$ if chronic respiratory failure

CONSIDER surgical treatments

11-33

CLUBBING
(HYPERTROPHIC PULMONARY OSTEOARTHROPATHY)

Def

A syndrome of bulbous enlargement of the terminal phalanges, arthritis, and periostitis due to overgrowth and inflammatory changes in the soft tissue.

Etiology

Primary cause unknown: Theories – hypoxia of local tissues, capillary stasis, chronic infections, A-V shunts.
Pulmonary: Alveolar proteinosis, chronic hypoxemia, pneumoconiosis, pulmonary infections, empyema, tumors, UIP.
Nonpulmonary: Bacterial endocarditis, CHD, hereditary, liver cirrhosis, long-term MV.
Unilateral clubbing: Local or aortic aneurysms, pulmonary hypertension with PDA..

CM

Skin-nail angle > 160°

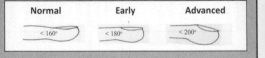

Normal	Early	Advanced
< 160°	< 180°	< 200°

COCCIDOIDOMYCOSIS	
Def	Systemic fungal infection characterized by caseating granulomas and its prevalence in the southwest USA.
Etiology	*Coccidioides immitis*, inhabits soil in semiarid regions. Most common source: dust storms, farming. **Route**: inhalation.
CM	Asymptomatic (majority) to death -- • Poorly localized chest pain aggravated by breathing • Nonproductive cough • Hemoptysis • Constitutional (other systems) symptoms. • Meningitis is common cause of death.
CXR	Nodules, cavitation, bronchopneumonia, hilar enlargement, pleural effusion.
Tx	• Anti-fungal drugs (amphotericin B), • Various azoles • Airway Clearance • Surgical for severe hemoptysis • BP fistula or persistent cavitary growth

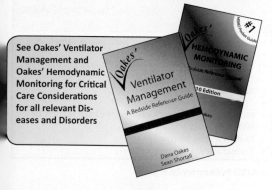

See Oakes' Ventilator Management and Oakes' Hemodynamic Monitoring for Critical Care Considerations for all relevant Diseases and Disorders

	CONGESTIVE HEART FAILURE HEART FAILURE
Def	Inability of the left ventricle to maintain adeq. CO, thereby failing to provide sufficient blood flow to meet the metabolic demands of the body. Usually LHF with/without RHF.
Etiology	Many and various – Arrhythmias, acquired or congenital HD, infection, ischemia, shock.
CM	**Cardiac:** ↑HR, murmurs (S3), ↓BP, peripheral edema, JVD, hepatomegaly **Respiratory:** ↑RR, dyspnea, othopnea, crackles/wheeze, hypoxemia, cough (pink, frothy), PND, pulsus alternans. **Other:** Fatigue, irritable, sweating
CXR	Cardiomegaly, ↑pulmonary vasculature? Kerly B lines
EBG	• ACC/AHA Guideline Update for the Diagnosis and Management of Chronic Heart Failure in the Adult • Chronic Heart Failure: Management of chronic heart failure in adults in primary and secondary care (NICE) • 2010 Heart Failure Society of America Comprehensive Heart Failure Practice Guideline
CC	• See Oakes' Hemodynamic Monitoring for detailed Cardiopulmonary Function • See Oakes' Ventilator Management for detailed Mechanical Ventilation Strategies
Tx	• Treat cause and complications (pulmonary edema) • O₂ therapy • ↑CO (↓afterload, adequate preload, ↑ myocardial contractility, prevent dysrhythmias) • Keep HOB > 10-45 degrees • Consider NPPV with adequate EPAP • Mechanical Ventilation with adequate PEEP to decrease WOB, unload LV • Restrict Intake, Diurese • Correct anemia and electrolytes

SEE ALSO Pulmonary Edema

	COR PULMONALE (RT HEART FAILURE, RHF)
Def	RV hypertrophy and dilatation caused by pulmonary disease
Etiology	**Pulmonary hypertension due to:** **Anatomical increase:** Vascular disease, diffuse interstitial fibrosis, granulomas, emphysema. **Vascular motor increase:** Hypoxemia, hypercarbia, acidosis. **Combined:** Multiple small pulmonary emboli. ↑ blood flow, volume, or viscosity (polycythemia). **Note:** Neither LHD nor CHD is included as a factor. **Acute cor pulmonale:** pulmonary embolism & ARDS.
CM	• Dyspnea • Cough • Chest discomfort • Hepatomegaly • Peripheral edema • JVD • Hypoxemia • Cyanosis • ↓$PaCO_2$ • ↑ Hematocrit • ECG Δ.
CXR	Right ventricular enlargement
CC	• See **Oakes' Hemodynamic Monitoring** for detailed Cardio-pulmonary Function • See **Oakes' Ventilator Management** for detailed Mechanical Ventilation Strategies
Tx	• Tx underlying lung disease • Reduce RV afterload • Relieve cause of pulmonary hypertension • O_2 therapy • Diuretics, calcium channel blockers, anticoagulants to reduce risk of blood clots

	CRYPTOCOCCOSIS
Def	Pulmonary fungal infection that can disseminate throughout the body
Etiology	Inhalation of *Cryptococcus neoformans* (G+ yeast) spores. Inhabits soil rich in pigeon droppings.
CM	Varies from asymptomatic (most common) to ARDS: • Cough with mucoid sputum • Hemoptysis • Pleuritic pain, • Dyspnea • Fever.
CXR	Multiple nodules or diffuse infiltrates, bronchopneumonia, occasional cavitation.
EBG	• Clinical Practice Guidelines for the Management of Cryptococcal Disease, 2010 Update by the Infectious Disease Society of America
Tx	Amphotericin B with/without flucytosine for several weeks, afterward oral fluconazole

	CUSHING'S SYNDROME
Def	Clinical syndrome characterized by the manifestations listed below.
Etiology	↑ Corticosteroids either by adrenal gland production or chronic iatrogenic administration.
CM	Fat deposition: moon face, buffalo hump, truncal obesity. Muscle weakness and fatigability, osteoporosis, diabetic mellitus, hypertension, emotional changes.

DIABETIC KETOACIDOSIS (DKA)

Def

Metabolic acidosis caused by accumulation of ketone bodies from tissue protein breakdown.

Respiratory Involvement: Significant Metabolic Acidosis will result in Respiratory Compensation (hyperventilation), with eventual tiring resulting in Respiratory Failure and a combined, sometimes significant Mixed Acidosis.

Etiology

- Insufficient insulin in known diabetes (or undiagnosed)
- Diagnostic Criteria (2009 ADA)

	Mild	Moderate	Severe
Plasma Glucose > 250 mg/dL			
Arterial pH	7.25 - 7.30	7.00-7.24	< 7.00
Serum HCO_3	15-18	10-14	< 10
Ketones (serum/urine)	+	+	+
Anion Gap	> 10	> 12	> 12
Mental Status	Alert	Drowsy	Stupor/ Coma
$PaCO_2$	Alkalosis	Alkalosis or Normal	Acidosis

CM

- Kussmaul breathing (↓ $PaCO_2$),
- Sweet breath odor (ketones)
- Vomiting, Headache, Dehydration
- ↓ Na+, ↓ K+,
- Coma, Long-Term Neurological disruption

EBG

- **American Diabetes Association Clinical Practice Recommendations 2009 Position Statement "Hyperglycemic Crises in Adult Patients with Diabetes"**

Tx

- Correct acidosis
- Fluid Infusions with careful consideration of electrolytes
- Careful glucose/insulin control and monitoring (give insulin once K+ deficiencies have been corrected. Administration of bicarb may further complicate K+ control)
- Support Respiratory status, as required

EMPHYSEMA	
Def	Enlargement and destruction of the air spaces beyond the terminal bronchiole.
Types	**Panlobular**: Affects alveoli, alveolar ducts and sacs **Alpha-1 Antitrypsin Deficiency** **Centribolular**: Affects respiratory bronchioles **Normal** **Centrilobular** **Panlobular** 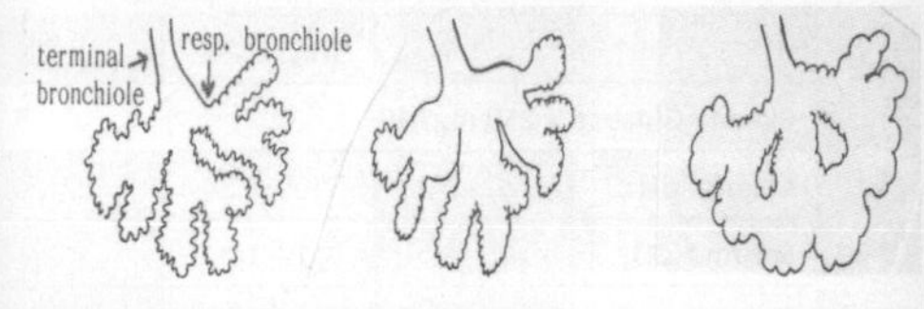
Etiology	**Panlobular**: constitutional defect, idiopathic, alpha-1 anti-trypsin (genetic) deficiency generally manifesting by the 4th to 5th decade **Centribolular**: Smoking, air pollution, chronic bronchitis, infection, occupational exposure to dusts
CM	See COPD
CXR	**See COPD**
EBG	• See ***ATS/ERS Statement: Standards for the Diagnosis and Management of Individuals with Alpha-1 Antitrypsin Deficiency*** at www.thoracic.org.
CC	• **See Oakes' Ventilator Management for Mechanical Ventilation Strategies**
Tx	**See COPD**

EMPYEMA	
Def	Purulent fluid in the pleural cavity.
Etiol	Extension of infection from pneumonia, lung abscess, sub-diaph. abscess, pneumothorax, trauma, bronchiectasis, TB
CM	Signs and symptoms of the infection, plus physical signs of fluid in the pleural cavity. See pleural effusion.
CXR	Fluid in the pleural space and or pleural thickening.
Tx	Chest tube drainage or surgery

FLAIL CHEST	
Def	Condition in which a portion of the chest wall moves in a direction opposite to the rest of the thorax. Instability due to fractures of two or more ribs in at least two locations.
Etiol	Chest trauma (usually mechanical such as in automobile crashes and industrial machinery accidents)
CM	Paradoxical movement of chest wall. Reduced ventilation to affected side, dyspnea, ↑WOB,, pain, splinting, atelectasis, hypoxemia. Usually accompanied by other pulmonary injuries.
CXR	Fractured ribs
CC	• See **Oakes' Ventilator Management** for Mechanical Ventilation Strategies
Tx	• Airway Clearance Therapies • Pain management to encourage deep breathing • If chest needs to be stabilized, use external fixation and Mechanical Ventilation (PEEP?)

GUILLIAN-BARRE' SYNDROME (GBS)

Def	Ascending muscular paralysis & profound autonomic dysfunction.
Etiology	Idiopathic, often follows recent flu-like infection. Autoimmune Rx?
CM	Ascending muscular weakness, pain, paralysis resulting in chest muscle and diaphragm paralysis and respiratory failure. Difficulty swallowing, possible aspiration. ↓ BP, ↓HR, bronchorrhea.
CC	• See **Oakes' Ventilator Management** for Mechanical Ventilation Strategies
Tx	Closely monitor pulmonary mechanics and airway control. Bronchial hygiene, & lung expansion to ↓ atelectasis, intubation/MV at VC ≈20 mL/kg and/or poor upper airway control.

HISTOPLASMOSIS

Def	Chronic systemic fungal infection characterized by prevalence in East Central USA and Mississippi Valley.
Etiology	*Histoplasma capsulatum*, inhabits soil rich with pigeon, bird, chicken, and bat droppings. **Route**: inhalation.
CM	Asymptomatic (majority) to fatal. Respiratory tract infection of varying severity. Dyspnea, chest pain, crackles, cough with scant mucoid sputum, constitutional symptoms.
CXR	Highly variable, cavitation, hilar calcification, widespread infiltrates.
EBG	**Clinical Practice Guidelines for the Management of Patients with Histoplasmosis, Update by the Infectious Diseases Society of America**
Tx	Anti-fungal drugs if severe.

HYPERSENSITIVITIY PNEUMONIA (ALLERGIC ALVEOLITIS)	
Def	Extrinsic allergic pneumonias occurring in workers sensitized to organic dusts.
Types	Bagassosis, bird-breeder's lung, farmer's lung, humidifier lung, etc.
Etiology	Organic dusts (bacteria, fungi, animal proteins, chemicals).
CM	Depends on antigen type, concentration, size, shape, patient sensitivity, length of time/amount of exposure. Dyspnea, cough, chest tightness, wheezing/crackles, tachypnea, hypoxemia, PFT's – restrictive, constitutional symptoms.
CXR	Varies with specific etiology. ↑ bronchovascular markings, diffuse finely modular shadows, hyperinflation, honeycombing.
Tx	Avoid antigens, treat symptoms, steroids for acute forms.

INFLUENZA	
Def	Acute respiratory tract viral infection characterized by the sudden onset of symptoms.
Etiology	Viral: influenza A, B, C
CM	Sudden onset of constitutional symptoms, plus rhinitis, pharyngitis, tracheitis, bronchitis, pneumonia.
Tx	Treat symptoms and complications

	INTERSTITIAL LUNG DISEASE (ILD) INTERSTITIAL PNEUMONIA
Def	A large variety (150) of diffuse pulmonary infiltrative disorders characterized by alveolar wall injury leading to the development of interstitial / alveolar exudates, hyaline membranes, and fibrosis.
Etiology	• Idiopathic pulmonary fibrosis (50%) • (Alveolar proteinosis, BOOP, DIP, Hamman -Rich, Sarcoidosis, ,UIP) • Chemical irritants • Collagen disorder's (Goodpastures, SLE) • Drug-induced (illicit or medications, O_2 toxicity, radiation therapy) • Familial disorders • Infections • Neoplasms • Prolonged circulatory failure • Occupational lung disease (See Hypersensitivity pneumonia, Pneumoconiosis)
CM	Varies with extent of involvement: • DOE (most common) • Cough (maybe productive) • Crackles • Clubbing/Fatigue • Hypoxemia leading to cor pulmonale • Respiratory alkalosis • PFTs-restrictive • Constitutional sympt.
CXR	Varies with stage, normal or reticulonodular densities or ground glass haziness and honeycombing
EBG	**The Official Statement of the ATS/ERS/JRS/ALAT: Idiopathic Pulmonary Fibrosis: Evidence-based Guidelelines for Diagnosis and Management**
Tx	Avoid exposure, O_2 therapy?, steroids?, cytotoxic agents?

SEE ALSO Hypersensitivity Pneumonia (Organic), Pneumoconiosis (Inorganic), and Sarcoidosis

KYPHOSCOLIOSIS

Def	Angulation of the vertebral column resulting in a restrictive chest wall disorder. **Kyphosis**: posterior curvature of the spine **Scoliosis**: lateral curvature of the spine
Etiology	Idiopathic (80%), congenital, bone TB, neuromuscular disorder.
CM	Marked chest asymmetry, marked variations in chest excursion and BS, DOE, ↓ Ccw, ↑ WOB, ↑ $PaCO_2$, hypoxemia leading to cor pulmonale, polycythemia, atelectasis, recurrent pulmonary infections, PFT's – restrictive.
CXR	Marked bone deformation, atelectasis..
CC	• See **Oakes' Ventilator Management** for Mechanical Ventilation Strategies
Tx	Spinal fixation, lung inflation therapy, bronchial hygiene.

LUNG ABSCESS

Def	Inflammatory necrotic lesion of the lung parenchyma that contains purulent material.
Etiology	Aspiration of oro/nasopharyngeal contents containing necrotic infectious organisms (usually anaerobes).
CM	Highly variable. Most common: periodic cough with expectoration of large amounts of purulent, fetid, bloody sputum. Dull chest pain, consolidation (dull to percussion), crackles, clubbing, ↓ BS, (maybe cavernous), constitutional symptoms.
CXR	Definitive diagnosis: rounded area of dense infiltration surrounding a radiolucent center which may present with a horizontal air-fluid interface.
Tx	Antibiotics, postural drainage.

LUNG CANCERS (LUNG CA)	
Def	A disease of uncontrolled cell growth in tissues of the lung, which may lead to metastasis beyond the lungs.
Types	Non-small cell lung cancer (NSCLC): 85%, adenocarcinoma (most common), squamous (epithelial) cell, large cell undifferentiated Small-cell lung cancer (SCLC), or Oat Cell Carcinoma: 15%, most aggressive
Etiology	**Primary cause:** 85% linked to smoking (COPD) **Secondary causes:** hereditary, racial, dietary, occupational/environmental exposure (air pollution, asbestos, radiation, radon).

CM

Asymptomatic to death, depending on type/stage of cancer. Stage is the extent the cancer has spread (metastasis and degree of lung involvement).

Persistent cough Chest pain/dyspnea	Hemoptysis Localized wheezing	Repeated infections Clubbing

Staging

IA: T1N0M0 IB: T2N0M0	IIA: T1N1M0 IIB: T2N1M0 T3N0M0	IIIA: T3N1M0 T(1-3)N2M0 IIIB: T4N(0-3)M0 T(1-4)N3M0	IV: T(any) N(any)M1

CXR	Atelectasis, rounded masses of variable size and shape, unilateral hilar enlargement, consolidation, pleural effusion. CAT and PET Scans provide type & location details
EBG	**Diagnosis and Management of Lung Cancer Executive Summary: ACCP Evidence-Based Clinical Practice Guidelines**
Tx	**Bronchoalveolar involvement**: smoking cessation therapy, O₂ therapy, lung inflation therapy, Airway Clearance Therapy, pulm rehab. **NSCLC**: Surgical resection is treatment of choice for early stage, chemotherapy for advanced stage **SCLC**: Chemotherapy with or without radiotherapy

MYOCARDIAL INFARCTION	
Def	Acute myocardial ischemia → necrosis of cardiac muscle
Etiology	↓ coronary artery perfusion resulting from coronary artery disease (atherosclerosis) or spasm; ventricular hypertrophy; hypoxia
CM	Dependent on location and extent of ischemic damage and resultant myocardial damage. Common findings: ↑ HR, chest pain (angina pectoris) /radiating pain (teeth, jaw, neck, shoulder, ↓ arm), SOB, orthopnea, nausea, diaphoresis, anxiety.
CC	• See Oakes' Hemodynamic Monitoring for greater details • See **Oakes' Ventilator Management** for Mechanical Ventilation Strategies
Tx	Limit infarct size (0₂ therapy), maintain optimal CO/tissue perfusion, bed rest, medications (anti-platelet [aspirin], anti-coagulants [heparin], anti-dysrhythmics, β-blockers, nitrates, morphine, ACE inhibitors.)

MYASTHENIA GRAVIS	
Def	Disorder of neuromuscular transmission of the voluntary (skeletal) muscles characterized by muscle weakness and easy fatigability, which often affects the respiratory muscles.
Etiology	Acquired auto-immune disorder. Note: A "myasthenic syndrome" sometimes accompanies sarcoidosis, hyper or hypothyroidism and lung cancer.
CM	Extreme weakness and fatigability, choking, aspiration, respiratory insufficiency. Diagnosed and temporary relief by anti-cholinesterase drugs (neostigmine bromide, edrophonium). **Myasthenic crisis**: acute event characterized by respiratory compromise. **Cholinergic crisis**: over-treatment of anti-cholinesterase (clinical presentation similar to a myasthenic crisis). **Note**: Tensilon test: Give edrophonium chloride – if myasthenic crisis, pt improves; if cholinergic crisis, pt worsens.
CC	• See **Oakes' Ventilator Management** for Mechanical Ventilation Strategies
Tx	Monitor pulmonary mechanics and airway control, anti-cholinesterase drugs, bronchial hygiene, MV, ACTH?, immunosuppressants?, steroids?, thymectomy?.

See Oakes' Ventilator Management and Oakes' Hemodynamic Monitoring for Critical Care Considerations for all relevant Diseases and Disorders

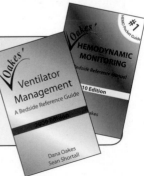

	NEAR-DROWNING
Def	Aspiration of water during submersion causing hypoxia and acidosis with survival for ≥ 24 hrs after submersion. **Drowning** = death by asphyxia < 24 hrs following submersion.
Types	Differences between fresh and salt water near drowning are theoretical, and have no clinical significance concerning patient mgmt. Water temperature and the presence of contaminants in the water are greater considerations than the salinity.
Etiology	Leaving small children unattended, trauma (head/neck), exhaustion, intoxication (alcohol, drugs), seizures.
CM	Variable with minimal findings to cardiorespiratory arrest (often a delay of 2-6 hrs). **Pulmonary**: cyanosis, pallor, crackles, frothy sputum, wheezing, cough, apnea. **Cerebral**: changed mental status, seizures, stupor, coma. **Other**: arrhythmias, evidence of trauma, metabolic acidosis, shock.
CXR	May be normal; atelectasis, pulmonary edema (alveolar & interstitial infiltrates)
Tx	CPR if needed, O_2 therapy ASAP, treat bronchospasm, treat hypothermia if present, treat respiratory failure with O_2, MV with PEEP, and HCO_3. Use PEEP early (especially if O_2 > 40%). Treat cerebral edema with diuretics and hyperventilation. Treat pulmonary edema ("secondary drowning") with diuretics and PFFP/CPAP. Watch for arrhythmias, inotropic drugs to improve tissue and cerebral perfusion? Antibiotics? (If infected source).

ORNITHOSIS (PSITTACOSIS, PARROT FEVER)	
Def	Atypical pneumonia transmitted to humans from birds
Etiology	Inhalation of gram-negative bacterium *Chlamydia psittaci*, which inhabits excrement of Psitticine birds (parrots, cockatoos, lorikeets) infected with *C. psittaci*.
CM	Asymptomatic to severe pneumonia. Cough with scanty, mucoid sputum progressing to mucopurulent, hemoptysis, dyspnea, tachypnea, hypoxemia (severe), chest pain, constitutional symptoms, respiratory failure
CXR	Variable, but may reveal patchy or lobar consolidation
Tx	Antibiotics (tertracycline, erythromycin) and bronchial hygiene

OXYGEN TOXICITY	
Def	Pulmonary and systemic damage and injury caused by prolonged inhalation of an elevated P_IO_2.
Etiology	**Pulmonary oxygen toxicity** (normobaric conditions): O_2 less than 40% may never show effects, 100% may show effects within 24 hrs. **CNS (systemic) oxygen toxicity** (hyperbaric conditions)
CM	**Pulmonary** - first-sign: symptoms of acute tracheobronchitis, substernal discomfort, dry hacking cough, vomiting, nausea, tachypnea, hypopnea, chest pain, then progressing to ARDS and pulmonary fibrosis. **CNS** - convulsions, nausea, dizziness, vision/hearing abnormalities, muscle twitching, anxiety, confusion, hiccups, fatigue.
CC	• See Oakes' Neonatal/Pediatric Respiratory Care for special considerations related to oxygenation in Neonates
Tx	Keep F_IO_2 less than 0.4 if possible.

PECTUS CARINATUM (PIGEON CHEST)

Def	Outward bending of the anterior ribs forcing sternum outward and increasing AP diameter (convex appearance)
Etiology	Congenital, ricketts, kyphoscoliosis, A or V septal defect.
CM	Usually asymptomatic; when symptomatic: decreased stamina/ endurance, frequent respiratory infections, chest pain.
Tx	Usually none; cosmetic or corrective surgery

PECTUS EXCAVATUM (FUNNEL CHEST)

Def	Posterior displacement of the lower sternum (concave appearance)
Etiology	Congenital
CM	Usually asymptomatic, unless severe, then ↓ stamina/endurance, cardiac palpitations during exercise; restrictive lung disease
CXR	Broadened cardiac silhouette
Tx	Usually none; cosmetic or corrective surgery

PLEURAL EFFUSION (HYDROTHORAX)

Def	Excessive accumulation of pleural fluid
Types	**Chylothorax**: chyle **Hemothorax**: blood **Hydrothorax**: serous fluid **Pyothorax**: pus
Etiology	**Transudation**: Plasma passing from vessels into pleural space due to hydraulic or osmotic abnormalities (↓ proteins, ↓ LDH). Causes: atelectasis, CHF, hypoproteinemia, lymphatic obstruction, liver cirrhosis, nephrotic syndrome, pericarditis. **Exudation**: Inflammatory effusion resulting from capillary damage or lymphatic blockage (↑ proteins, ↑ LDH). Causes: acute pancreatitis, cancer, drugs, infections (TB), post-MI syndrome, pulmonary embolism, rheumatoid arthritis, sarcoidosis, SLE. **Note**: See empyema
CM	Dependent on amount of fluid: dyspnea, cough, pain, ↑RR, orthopnea, ↓ BS, egophony, ↓ fremitus, dull to percussion (on affected side), progressing to tracheal deviation and CV compromise with massive effusion > 300 mL.
CXR	Radiopacity of involved cavity and blunting of costophrenic angle, mediastinal shift.
Tx	Depends on size of effusion and symptomology: • If small and/or minimal symptoms, may just be observed • Oxygen Therapy, as needed • Treat underlying cause (see causes above in Etiology) • Thoracentesis or Thoracostomy Tube • Pleurodesis* (malignancy) • Shunt

*Pleurodesis is the process by which a chemical or medication is inserted between 2 layers of pleura, causing them to adhere to each other, with the goal of preventing recurring pleural effusions.

PLEURITIS (PLEURISY)

Def	Inflammation of the pleura
Etiology	Bacterial or viral pneumonia, pleural effusion, pneumothorax, pulmonary emboli, SLE, neoplasms, pulmonary abscess, TB
CM	Abrupt onset; sharp, stabbing pain aggravated by insp. or cough, often unilateral + localized, SOB, intercostal tenderness, splinting, pleural friction rub, infection evid. (if cause).
CXR	Thickening of pleura
Tx	Correct underlying cause

PNEUMOCONIOSIS

Def	Lung disease caused by inhalation of inorganic dust &/ or chemical fumes (See also Hypersensitivity pneumonia: organic).
Etiology	Type of inorganic dust Nonreactive dust: coal (coal-workers lung, black lung) tin, iron (siderosis) barium (baritosis), cement, antimony, titanium Fibrogenic dust (nodular): silica (silicosis), aluminum or magnesium silicate Diffuse: asbestos fibers (asbestosis), aluminum oxide, beryllium, hard metals
CM	Asymptomatic to death – Dependent on type and concentration of dust/fumes, host susceptibility, length of exposure, deposition factors, particle size.
CC	• **See Oakes' Ventilator Management (Restrictive Disorders) for Mechanical Ventilation Strategies**
Tx	Avoid causative agent, treat symptoms, O_2 therapy, bronchodilators, steroids

PNEUMOCYSTIS PNEUMONIA (PCP, PNEUMOCYSTOSIS)	
Def	Pneumonia caused by the organism *P. jirovecii*, primarily occurring in immunocompromised patients. See AIDS.
Etiology	*Pneumocystis jirovecii* (a fungus); contagious and acquired by patients with depressed cellular immunity or antibody formation from asymptomatic carriers. (Previously called P. carinii)
CM	Slow progression to severe dyspnea and tachypnea, cyanosis, anxiety, concurrent bacterial infection is common, dry cough, fever, PFTs – restrictive.
CXR	Massive consolidation spreading from hilar through most of lung.
EBG	**Official ATS Workshop Summary: Recent Advances and Future Directions in Pneumocystis Pneumonia (PCP)**
Tx	Trimethoprim-sulfamethoxazole (TMP-SMZ), atovaquone, pentamidine, antiretroviral therapy, corticosteroids, O_2 therapy, MV.

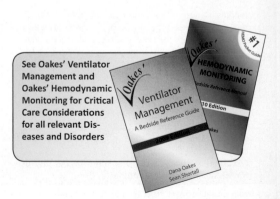

See Oakes' Ventilator Management and Oakes' Hemodynamic Monitoring for Critical Care Considerations for all relevant Diseases and Disorders

PNEUMONIAS (PNA)

Def	Inflammatory process of the lung's air spaces. Diagnosed by CXR infiltrate, plus 2 or more of: fever, ↑ WBC, &/or purulent sputum.
Types	**Lobar** – Air-space inflammation often affecting entire lobe. **Broncho** – Inflammation of alveoli and contiguous bronchi **Interstitial** – Pneumonitis

Etiology

Causes:

• Aspiration • Bacterial (TB) • Fungal • Hypersensitivity • Viral	See each type for more specifics

Sources:

Healthcare-Associated	HCAP	• Any Pt hospitalized 2+ days within 90 days of infection • Received recent IV Antibiotics, Chemotherapy, or wound care within past 30 days of infection • Attended hospital or hemodialysis Clinic
Hospital Acquired	HAP	• PNA that occurs > 48 hrs after admission (not incubating at admission)
Ventilator Associated	VAP	• PNA that occurs > 48-72 hrs after endotracheal intubation
Community Acquired	CAP	• Those not meeting any of the above definitions

EBG

IDSA/ATS Consensus Guidleines on the Management of Community-Acquired Pneumonia in Adults at www.thoracic. org.

ATS Guidelines for the Management of Adults with Hospital-Acquired, Ventilator-associated, and Healthcare-associated Pneumonia at www.thoracic.org.

PNEUMOTHORAX (& AIR LEAK SYNDROME)

Def	Accumulation of gas in the pleural space or other thoracic areas, usually with associated lung collapse	
Types	**Spontaneous**	no obvious causative event - spont. rupture of bleb/bullae on viseral pleura
	1°	no identifiable lung disease
	2°	pre-existing lung disease
	Traumatic	Includes Iatrogenic and Other
	Indirect	Barotrauma (excessive pressure), often as a result of mechanical ventilation (esp in presence of reduced compliance)
	Direct	Related to Rib fx, surgery, thoracentesis, Line insertions, tracheostomy, etc.
	Tension	Pneumothorax of any cause where air leaks into the pleural cavity, but can't escape - "one-way valve" resulting in a pressure > atmospheric during breathing cycle – **acute medical emergency**.
	Pneumo-Pericardium	Accumulation of gas in the pericardial sac
	Pneumo-Mediastinum	Accumulation of gas in the mediastinum
Etiology	• BP fistula • Cancer • COPD • Necrotizing pneumonia • Tuberculosis • Spontaneous or traumatic (See below).	

CM	Asymptomatic to sudden onset of dyspnea, anxiety, ↑RR, ↑ HR, cyanosis, hypoxemia, pleuritic pain (sharp), subcut. emphysema, ↑A-a gradient **Both tension & non-tension:** ↓BS, ↓fremitus, hyperresonance, enlarged hemithorax with ↓ chest expansion (all same side). **Tension:** tympany (same side), mediastinal/tracheal shift (opposite side), severe CV compromise, JVD. **Clinically stable:** RR < 24/min, HR 60-120/min, BP normal, SaO_2 > 90%, patient can speak in whole sentences between breaths. (unstable = lacking these characteristics)
CXR	Air in pleural space or mediastinum, ↑ radiolucency, lung collapse (towards hilar on affected side), absent bronchovascular markings Tracheal/mediastinal shift away from affected side and flattened diaphragm, if tension. **Small spontaneous** = < 3 cm apex-to-cupola **Large spontaneous** = > 3 cm apex-to-cupola
EBG	Management of Spontaneous Pneumothorax, American College of Chest Physicians Delphi Consensus Statement
CC	• See **Oakes' Ventilator Management** for in-depth information on pneumothoraces, particularly Barotrauma • See **Oakes' Neonatal/Pediatric Respiratory Care** for in-depth information on Air Leak Syndromes including barotrauma

Tx	Tension pneumothorax requires
	an EMERGENT THORACENTESIS
	
	Spontaneous pneumothorax:
	Clinically stable with small pneumothorax:
	   1°: observe
	   2°: observe and/or aspirate or chest tube
	Clinically stable with large pneumothorax:
	   2°: re-expand lung with catheter or chest tube
	Clinically unstable with any size pneumothorax:
	   2°: re-expand lung with catheter or chest tube
	Recurrent pneumothorax:
	   Thoracoscopy, pleurodesis, or bullectomy

PULMONARY EDEMA (CARDIAC ASTHMA)

Def	Accumulation of vascular fluid in alveoli or pulmonary interstitium
Types	Interstitial – Fluid moves only into the interstitium Alveolar – Fluid moves into the interstitium, plus the alveoli.

Etiology	**High-pressure pulmonary edema** (cardiogenic, hydrostatic)	**Permeability pulmonary edema** (non-cardiogenic, neurogenic)
	Transudation: due to a volume/ pressure overload of the pulmonary circulation *Causes*: acute MI, arrhythmias, CHF, infection, hypervolemia, LVF, renal failure, shock, valve disease	*Exudation*: due to an ↑permeability of the pulmonary capillary membrane. *Causes*: ARDS, CNS (hemorrhage, trauma, stroke, tumors, ↑ ICP), near drowning, smoke inhalation, O_2 toxicity

CM	Varies with severity of underlying disorder (↑severity as ↑ fluid). **General**: Sudden anxiety, restlessness, orthopnea, cyanosis, hypoxemia, diaphoresis **Resp**: ↑ RR, dyspnea, cough (dry to pink, frothy fluid), basal crackles/wheezing, SOB, PND, ↓ C **CV**: ↑ HR, ↓ BP, cold clammy skin, JVD, peripheral edema (See also page 1-17 and 8-12)
CXR	**Interstitial**: Haziness of vasculature and hilar **Alveolar**: Irregular, poorly defined ascinar shadows forming a "butterfly" or "bat wing" pattern. **Both**: Disparity between upper and lower lobe venous calibers. LVH when due to CHF. Air-bronchograms
CC	• See **Oakes' Ventilator Management** for Mechanical Ventilation Strategies • See **Oakes' Hemodynamic Monitoring** for further information on cardiopulmonary function
Tx	Treat underlying cause. O_2 as needed, diuretics, inotropes and afterload reducing agents, morphine, CPAP, BIPAP, MV with PEEP, cardioversion/resuscitation if needed.

PULMONARY EMBOLISM (PULMONARY INFRACTION)

Def	Blockage of part of pulmonary vascular bed by blood-borne material, sometimes causing pulmonary infarction (necrosis).

Etiology	**Blood (clots, thrombi)(90%):**
	   Blood stasis – bedrest, CHF, obesity, pregnancy, birth-control pills, post-op
	   Vessel wall abnorm.: trauma, phlebitis, infection/parasites
	   Abnormal blood coagulation – ↑ clotting or ↓ lysis of clots
	Air - CVP line placement
	Fat (bone marrow) -fractures, esp. leg bones
	Foreign material - drug abuse, indwelling catheters, tumors

CM

EBM suggests using a validated prediction scoring system before proceeding with testing for PE. Wells Scoring System and Revised Geneva Scoring System are common.

Revised Geneva Scoring System, Summarized

Risk Factors	Age > 65 y		1
	Previous DVT or PE		3
	General Anes. or Fx of ↓ Extrem in last month		2
	Acute malignant condition		2
Sympt.	Unilateral lower limb pain		3
	Hemoptysis		2
Clinical	HR 75-94		3
	HR > 95		5
	Pain on lower limb and Unilateral edema		4

Low (0-3), Intermediate (4-10), High (11+)

General	Sudden anxiety, orthopnea, restlessness, cyanosis, possibly leg swelling and pain
Respiratory	dyspnea & sharp chest pain (two most common), ↑ RR, cough (nonproductive to hemoptysis), crackles, wheeze, friction rub,↓ BS, splinting, PFTs – restrictive
CV	↑HR, hypoxemia leading to cor pulmonale

CXR	Often normal. May have ↑ pulmonary artery size, abrupt tapering of occluded artery, consolidation (atelectasis or infarction), line shadows.
EBG	**Current Diagnosis of Venous Thromboembolism in Primary Care, American Academy of Physicians and American College of Physicians**
CC	See **Oakes' Hemodynamic Monitoring** for detailed cardiopulmonary function aspects
Tx	<ul><li>Prophylaxis</li><li>O2 therapy</li><li>Treat anxiety/pain</li><li>Anticoagulant therapy (heparin & warfarin)</li><li>Fibrinolytic therapy (alteplase & reteplase)</li><li>Blood Type: Thrombolytic therapy (urokinase & streptokinase)</li><li>Fat Type: Steroids</li><li>Embolectomy?</li></ul>

	RESPIRATORY FAILURE **(ACUTE RESPIRATORY FAILURE, ARF)**
Def	Inability of the respiratory system to maintain normal O_2 uptake and CO_2 removal, i.e., failure to maintain gas exchange.
Types	**Hypoxemic**: Type I, lung failure, oxygenation failure, or respiratory insufficiency. **Hypercapnic**: Type II, pump failure, or ventilatory failure.
Etiology	Any disease or disorder which compromises the ability of the lungs to provide sufficient O_2/CO_2 exchange.

	Hypoxemic	**Hypercapnic**
CM	$PaO_2 < 60$ mm Hg on FiO_2 $\geq .50$ or $PaO_2 < 40$ mm Hg (any FiO_2) $SaO_2 < 90\%$; Plus, signs and symptoms of hypoxemia (see O_2 Therapy, Chapter 10)	Acute ↑ in $PaCO_2 > 50$ mm Hg with concurrent ↓ in pH < 7.30 (or $PaCO_2$ acutely above baseline in CO_2 retainers) Plus, signs and symptoms of hypercapnia (see Oakes' ABG Pocket Guide)

CC	Complete critical care coverage of Respiratory Failure can be found in Oakes' Ventilator Management
Tx	Both: Treat underlying cause , O_2 therapy, NPPV or MV, fluid and nutritional management

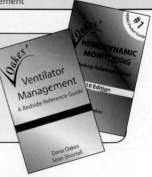

See Oakes' Ventilator Management and Oakes' Hemodynamic Monitoring for Critical Care Considerations for all relevant Diseases and Disorders

RESTRICTIVE LUNG DISEASE (DISORDER)

Def	Disease/disorder characterized by a ↓lung volumes/capacities
Etiology	**Parenchymal conditions:** 　Compression - fibrosis, pleural effusion, pneumothorax, tumor 　Infiltration - edema, infection, secretions, hyaline membranes 　Loss of volume - atelectasis, ARDS, ↓surfactant, lobectomy 　Replacement -fibrous tissue, tumors, etc **Chest wall abnorm.** – musculoskeletal/neuromusc. disorders **Nervous system control** – depression of drive, paralysis
CM	Dyspnea, hypoxemia leading to cor pulmonale, polycythemia, cyanosis, respiratory alkalosis/acidosis (late). ↓ lung volumes (VC ↓ more then FRC and RV), ↓C, normal flows (FEV₁, FVC)
Tx	Treat underlying disease

SARCOIDOSIS

Def	Relatively benign multisystem, chronic non-caseating granulomatous disorder of undetermined etiology.
Etiol	Unknown
CM	Asymptomatic to death. Primarily affects the lungs. Dyspnea, severe cough, scanty mucoid sputum, hypoxemia leading to cor pulmonale, respiratory alkalosis, crackles, constitutional symptoms, spontaneous pneumothorax, PFTs –restrictive.
CXR	Varies greatly
Tx	Tx symptoms, steroids to reduce inflammation; avoid calcium-rich food, vitamin D, sunlight, dusts, chemicals, and fumes

SEVERE ACUTE RESPIRATORY SYNDROME (SARS)	
Def	A contagious, severe respiratory illness (pneumonia) caused by a coronavirus, called SARS-associated coronavirus (SARS-CoV).
CM	Asymptomatic to death. Initial symptoms are flu-like; fever >100.4°F (>38°C), myalgia, sore throat, clinical findings of respiratory illness (dry cough, SOB, difficulty breathing, +/or hypoxia), and potentially evidence of pneumonia, or respiratory distress syndrome
CXR	Patchy, interstitial infiltrates, possible consolidation.
Tx	Respiratory isolation, no specific treatment recommendations at this time; treat symptoms, acquired pneumonia, and any respiratory failure.

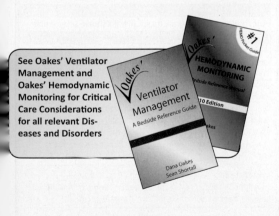

See Oakes' Ventilator Management and Oakes' Hemodynamic Monitoring for Critical Care Considerations for all relevant Diseases and Disorders

SHOCK

Def	Inadequate tissue perfusion resulting in hypoxic insult and causing widespread abnormal cell metabolism and membrane dysfunction.
Types	**Anaphylactic** – Systemic allergic rx causing circulatory failure **Cardiogenic** – Systemic hypoperfusion due to heart failure **Hypovolemic** – ↓ effective circulating volume (most common) **Neurogenic** – Sympathetic NS dysfunction resulting in massive peripheral vasodilation or hypoperfusion **Septic** (vasogenic) – Relative hypovolemia caused by any infection.

Etiology

Anaphylactic	Cardiogenic	Hypovolemic
Anesthetics, blood, drugs, foods, pollens, venoms	Acute MI, severe hypoxemia, arrhythmias, post-op failure, tension pneumothorax, valve dysfunction	Burns, dehydration, hemorrhage, sepsis, trauma

Neurogenic:

Anesthesia, brain trauma, drugs, insulin shock, severe pain

Septic (Systemic Inflammatory Response Syndrome – SIRS)

Acute pancreatitis, major trauma (including burns) hospital-acquired gram-negative bacilli or gram-positive cocci, fungal infection, immunoincompetence

CM	Varies according to etiology. Diaphoresis, cool clammy, moist skin, agitation, confusion, skin appears gray, dusky, or cyanotic, peripheral pulse rapid & weak, prolonged capillary refilling time, rapid shallow breathing, low to no urine output, chest pain, dizziness, unconsciousness
EBG	**Evidence-Based Guidelines** Available for Topic (Guidelines can be researched independently, or find direct links to information on RespiratoryUpdate.com)
CC	See **Oakes' Hemodynamic Monitoring** for detailed cardiopulmonary function aspects
Tx	Correct primary problem, O$_2$ and ventilation as needed, optimize CO and tissue perfusion.

SLEEP APNEAS

Def	Frequent cessation of breathing during sleep for ≥10 sec.

	Obstructive (OSA)	Central (CSA)
Types	Anatomic obstruction of upper airway. Ventilatory efforts continue.	Cessation of inspiratory efforts.
	Mixed – Combination of OSA and CSA.	
Etiology	Obesity, micrognathia, macroglossia, tonsillar hypertrophy, small or unstable pharynx	Exact etiology unknown; contributing conditions: CHF, stroke, brain lesions, cerebrovascular diseases
CM	Snoring and apnea with increasingly desperate efforts to inhale. May awaken gasping for air. PFTs-obstructive	Mild snoring and apnea
	BOTH: Daytime somnolence, memory loss, personality changes, depression, inability to concentrate, decreased mental acuity, potential arrhythmias, pulmonary hypertension.	
CXR	May develop RHF or LHF	
Tx	Polysomnography (see AARC CPG), avoid sleeping supine, avoid alcohol, sedatives, and REM inhibitors. O2 therapy as needed.	
	CPAP, BIPAP, tongue retainer, weight reduction, surgery	Pressure ventilation (time cycled) Negative pressure ventilation? Phrenic nerve pacemaker?

	SMOKE INHALATION (PULMONARY BURNS)
Def	Inhalation of smoke, fumes, or caustic agents into the tracheo-bronchial tree with potential tissue injury due to heat or toxins.
CM	**Signs and Symptoms of Respiratory Tract Injury** Facial burns, singed nasal hairs, reddened pharynx, hoarseness, cough, soot deposits, sooty sputum, central cyanosis, crackles, wheezes, stridor. Bronchoscopy is gold std for diagnosis. SpO2 can be profoundly inaccurate in the presence of increased HbCO levels - smoke inhalation. (See CO poisoning) **Stages** Stage I – Acute respiratory distress (wheezing/stridor, ↑RR, hoarseness, cough), may occur in a few hrs, resembles upper airway obstruction Stage II – Pulmonary edema (8-36 hrs) Stage III – Bacterial pneumonia (2 days – 3 weeks after injury)
CXR	**Variable**: Normal (Stage I), Pulmonary edema/ARDS (Stage II), Infiltrates (Stage 3)
CC	• See **Oakes' Ventilator Management** for Mechanical Ventilation Strategies
Tx	**Begin 100% O2 to all patients** (hyperbaric if CO poison), ensure adequate airway, laryngoscopy or bronchoscopy, closely monitor VS and I&O, , vigorous bronchial hygiene, bronchodilators - racemic epi?, pain meds?, corticosteroids?, Interpercussive Ventilation (IPV) **Burns to face, neck, oropharynx are all indicators to consider early intubation (airway swelling may not appear immediately following insult, but is likely to progress quickly once process begins)** **Treat complications:** ARDS, burns, pul edema, pneumonia, respiratory failure, shock

TRACHEAL-ESOPHAGEAL FISTULA (T-E FISTULA)	
Def	Abnormal passage between trachea and esophagus
Etiology	Often congenital, can be iatrogenic

CM	Three C's — Choking, Coughing, Cyanosis
	  Excess salivation, aspiration
	  Gastric distention

Tx	• NPO — Provide parenteral nutrition • Position Patient for patent airway and optimum ventilation • Aspirate secretions from oropharynx and pouch • Prevent aspiration • Surgical correction

See **BP Fistula** in Oakes' Ventilator Management

TRACHEO-INNOMINATE FISTULA (T-I FISTULA)	
Def	Abnormal passage between trachea and innominate artery
Etiology	Most likely complication from tracheostomy
CM	Bleeding from trach (should inspect quickly) Signs/Symptoms of Shock (see Shock)
Tx	• **This is a Life-Threatening Medical Emergency** • Inspect via Bronchoscopy - URGENT • Either overinflate cuff or digitally compress (with finger) • Surgical Intervention (rapid) • Very often is fatal

TUBERCULOSIS (TB)

Def	Chronic necrotizing bacterial infection, characterized by the formation of tubercles in the lung.
Types	**Miliary TB** - hematogenous disssem. throughout the body.
Etiology	*Mycobacterium tuberculosis*. Inhalation of droplet nuclei. *Predisposing factors*: malnutrition, diabetes, immunosuppression, HIV, CA, drug/etoh abuse, general debil., steroids
CM	Asymptomatic (majority) to death. Cough with mucoid or mucopurulent sputum, hemoptysis, chest tightness with dull pain, dyspnea, fatigue, fever, irritability, crackles/wheezes/bronchial BS, constitutional symptoms.
CXR	Variable with stage and type, often apical infiltrates with cavities.
EBG	**Evidence-Based Guidelines for the Evaluation, Treatment and Management of TB from WHO, ATS, CDC, and IDSA**
Tx	Use AIRBORNE Precautions, including a Negative-Pressure containment area. Anti-tuberculin drugs (Isoniazid, rifampin, pyrazinamide, ethambutol, streptomycin)

VIRAL PNEUMONIA

Def	Pneumonia caused by viruses
Etiology	Most all types. Esp. influenza, adeno, respiratory syncytial, and parainfluenza. *Mycoplasma pneumoniae*: viral like organism (use respiratory isolation), most common cause of nonbacterial pneumonia.
CM	Prior URI, dry cough, fever, DOE, cyanosis, fatigue, sore throat
CXR	Variable
Tx	Treat symptoms, if severe, treat like ARDS; bed rest, hydration

12 PHARMACOLOGY

CONTENTS

PHARM

!

Always check *manufacturers' inserts for changes in drug information to include dosages, indications, warnings, precautions and contraindications.*

This table is not all-inclusive, and dosages listed are adult dosages, unless indicated. Adult dose is often suitable for children > 12 years of age or > 40kg.

See Oakes' Ventilator Management for detailed information on Critical Care Drugs, including Diuretics, Anticoagulants, Paralytics and Paralytic-Reversal Drugs

Oakes'
Ventilator
Management
A Bedside Reference Guide

Dana Oakes
Sean Shortall

RESPIRATORY MEDICATION INDEX (PAGE FOUND IN CHAPTER)

Anti-Asthma	
Mast-Cell Stabilizers (14)	• **cromolyn Na**
Anti-Leukotrienes (15)	• **montelukast** (Singular) • **zafirlukast** (Accolate) • **zileuton** (Zyflo)

Bronchodilators	
SABA (16)	• **albuterol** (Accuneb, ProAir-Proventil, Ventolin, Vospire) • **levalbuterol** (Xopenex) • **pirbuterol acetate** (Maxair)
LABA (18)	• **arformoteral tartrate** (Brovana) • **formoterol fumarate** (Foradil, Perforomist) • **salmeterol** (Serevent) • **indacaterol maleate** (Arcapta)
Anti-Cholinergics (20)	• **aclidinium bromide** • **ipratropium bromide** (Atrovent) • **tiotropium bromide** (Spiriva)
Xanthines (21)	• **aminophylline**

Alpha-1 Antitrypsin (22)
• **alpha-1 proteinase inhibitor**

Anti-Infectives (23)
• **aztreonam** (Cayston) • **colistimethate Na** (Coly-Mycin) • **pentamidine isethionate** (Nebupent) • **ribavirin** (Virazole) • **tobramycin** (Tobi) • **zanamivir** (Relenza)

Cystic Fibrosis TransMembrane Conductance Regulator (CFTR) Potentiator (26)
• **ivacaftor** (Kalydeco)

IgE Blockers (27)
• **omalizumab** (Xolair)

PHARM

Mucoactives (27)

- **acetylcysteine** (Mucomyst, Mucosol)
- **dornase alfa-DNase** (Pulmozyme)

Inhaled Analgesics (28)

- **lidocaine**
- **morphine sulfate**

Inhaled Epinephrine (29)

- **racemic epinephrine** (S2, Primatine)

Phosphodiesterase Inhibitors (30)

- **roflumilast** (Daliresp)

Pulmonary Vasodilator (30)

- **Iloprost** (Ventavis) and others

Smoking Cessation (31)

• **varenicline** (Chantix)	• **Nicotrol patch** (Nicoderm CQ)
• **bupropion** (Zyban)	• **Nicorette Gum** (Commit Loz.)
• **nasal spray** (Nicotrol NS)	• **Nicotrol Oral Inhaler**

Steroids (34)

- **beclomethasone** (QVAR)
- **budesonide** (Pulmicort Turbuhaler, Pulmicort Respules)
- **ciclesonide** (Alvesco)
- **fluticasone** (Flovent)
- **mometasone furoate** (Asmanex)

Wetting Agents (34)

- **water**
- **saline** (hypotonic, isotonic, hypertonic)

Corticosteroid & LABA (35)

- **budesonide & formoterol** (Symbicort)
- **fluticasone and salmeterol** (Advair)
- **mometazone and formoterol** (Dulera)

Anti-Cholinergic and SABA (36)

- **ipratropium bromide & albuterol** (Combivent, Duoneb)

Abbreviations used in Prescriptions

Aa, aa	of each	IM	intra-muscular	Qid	4x/day
ac	before meals	IV	intra-vascular	Q2h	every 2 hours
ad	to, up to	I&O	intake & output	q3h	every 3 hours
ad lib	as much as needed	L	liter/left	q4h	every 4 hours
aq dist	distilled H2O	m	mix	qs, QS	as much as required
bid	2x/day	mixt	mixture	qt	quart
c̄	with	mL	milliliter	Rx	take
caps	capsule	nebul	spray	s	without
dil	dilute	non rep	not to be repeated	sig	write
el, elix	elixir	NPO	nothing by mouth	sol	solution
emuls	emulsion	ol	oil	solv	dissolve
et	and	p̄	after	sos	if needed (1x)
ext	extract	part acq	equal parts	ss	half
fl, fld	fluid	pc	after meals	stat	immediately
Ft, ft	make	po	by mouth	syr	syrup
gel	gel, jelly	prn	as needed	tab	tablet(s)
g, gm	gram	rect	rectally	tid	3x/day
gr	grain	pulv	powder	tinct	tincture
gtt	drop/drip	q	every	ung	ointment
ht	hypodermic tablet	qh	every hour	ut dict	as directed

Note: JCAHO has come out with an official "Do Not Use" list. The following chart lists excluded abbreviations, symbols and acronyms along with recommended and accepted terms or abbreviations to use.

Check JCAHO.org for updates

Medication Abbreviation Do-Not-Use List

Excluded Abbreviations	Recommendation
qd, QD	daily
qod, QOD	every other day
U, IU	Unit, International Unit
cc	mL, ml or milliliters
QN	every night, nightly
Q HS	Use "HS" of "at bedtime"
µg	micrograms or mcg
trailing zero, as in 1.0 mg	write 1 mg
No leading zero, as in .1mg	write 0.1 mg
degree sign for hours	spell out "hours"
/ when used in a handwritten prescription or order	spell out "per"
MS, MSIR, MSO4	write "morphine"
MgSO4	write "magnesium sulfate"
ZnSO4	write "zinc sulfate"
Apothecary symbol (e.g. grains)	write metric symbol (e.g. mg)
ss	spell out "sliding scale" or 1/2
per os	use "by mouth," "orally," or "PO"
D/C	Use discharge
Roman Numerals	Use arabic (4,100, etc.)
> and <	Use "greater than" or "less than"
sq or sub q	use subcut

Percentage Concentration of Solutions (weight to volume)

%	Ratios	g/L	g/100mL	g/mL	mg/100mL	mg/mL
100	1:1	1000	100	1	100,000	1000
10	1:10	100	10	0.1	10,000	100
5	1:20	50	5	0.05	5,000	50
1	1:100	10	1	0.01	1,000	10
0.5	1:200	5	0.5	0.005	500	5
0.1	1:1000	1	0.1	0.001	100	1

Medication Adminisration Procedures

Every time you administer medications, you should be following these procedures:

1. Review patient chart, verifying doctor's orders, code status, allergies, etc.
2. Assure you have the **right medication**.
3. Assure you have the **right dose** (including concentration).
4. Assure you have the **right time**.
5. Assure you have the **right route** (MDI vs. DPI vs. Neb).
6. Verify **right patient** (check I.D. bracelet, DOB).
7. Complete an adequate pre-, mid-, and post assessment.
8. See Mixing and Compatability Guide for commonly used aerosolized medications at RespiratoryUpdate.com

Major Red Flag Drugs

(high potential for Drug-Drug interactions)

• Aspirin	• Theophylline
• Cimetidine	• Warfarin
• Penytoin	

Solving Dosage of Liquids, Tablets, and Capsules

1. Convert all measurements to the same unit
2. $\dfrac{\text{Original Strength}}{\text{Amount Supplied}} = \dfrac{\text{Desired Strength (dosage)}}{\text{Unknown amount to be supplied}}$

Example 1: How many mL of a drug must be given to deliver 75,000 units (50,000 units/mL)?	Example 2: How many mLs of a drug, at a concent. of 25 mg/mL of solution, would be needed to provide 100 mg?
$\dfrac{50,000}{\text{mL}} = \dfrac{75,000}{\text{X mL}}$	$\dfrac{25 \text{ mg}}{\text{mL}} = \dfrac{100 \text{ mg}}{\text{X mL}}$
$X = \dfrac{75,000}{50,000} = 1.5 \text{ mL}$	$X = \dfrac{100\text{mg}}{25 \text{ mg}} = 4 \text{ mL}$

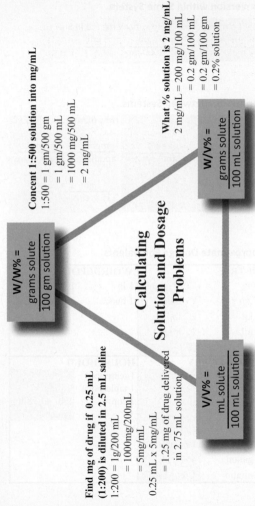

Calculating Solution and Dosage Problems

Concent 1:500 solution into mg/mL

1:500 = 1 gm/500 gm
= 1 gm/500 mL
= 1000 mg/500 mL
= 2 mg/mL

What % solution is 2 mg/mL

2 mg/mL = 200 mg/100 mL
= 0.2 gm/100 mL
= 0.2 gm/100 gm
= 0.2% solution

$$W/W\% = \frac{grams\ solute}{100\ gm\ solution}$$

$$W/V\% = \frac{grams\ solute}{100\ mL\ solution}$$

$$V/V\% = \frac{mL\ solute}{100\ mL\ solution}$$

Find mg of drug if 0.25 mL (1:200) is diluted in 2.5 mL saline

1:200 = 1g/200 mL
= 1000mg/200mL
= 5mg/mL
0.25 mL x 5mg/mL
= 1.25 mg of drug delivered in 2.75 mL solution

1 mL H20 = 1 gm H20 (spec gravity 1.0)   1 gm = 1,000 mg

12-7

Conversion within Same System

Set up a proportion:	How many mg are in 5 g?
$\dfrac{gm}{mg} = \dfrac{gm}{mg}$	$\dfrac{1\ gm}{1000\ mg} = \dfrac{5\ gm}{X}$

Conversion between Systems

Set up a proportion:	How many grains in 5 g?
$\dfrac{one\ system}{other\ system} = \dfrac{one\ system}{other\ system}$	$\dfrac{metric}{apothecary} = \dfrac{metric}{apothecary}$
	$\dfrac{1\ gm}{15\ grains} = \dfrac{5\ gm}{X}$

Approximate Dosage Equivalents

METRIC		AVOIRDUPOIS	
1 mg	0.015 grain	1 lb	454 gm
1 gm	15 grains	1 ounce	28.4 gm
1 kg	2.2 lbs		
1 mL	16 drops (gtts)		
APOTHECARY		**HOUSEHOLD**	
1 grain	60 mg	1 teaspoon	5 mL
1 ounce	30 gm	1 tablespoon	15 mL
1 fl ounce	30 mL	1 cup	240 mL, 8 fl ounces
1 pint	500 mL		
1 quart	1000 mL		
1 gallon	4000 mL		
1 minim	1 drop (gtt)		

!

Adjusting for Pediatric Dosages

Remember that recommended dosages are only estimates. Dosages should be individualized - adjust for variations in maturity, metabolism, temperature, obesity, edema, illness and individual tolerances.

Current literature supports BSA as the most consistent and accurate method of drug dosing over a wide range of body sizes. However, for small children (< 10 kg) dosing should be made on a mg/kg basis as BSA increases disproportionately as weight decreases.

Most drugs are dosed on a mg/kg basis in children. Due to differences in distribution, metabolism, and elimination, children require higher mg/kg dose than adults. While this works well for younger children, in older larger children and adolescents (>40 kg), when dosed by this method, adult doses can often be exceeded.

For this reason:

**never give a child a dose greater
than the usual adult dose,
regardless of height or weight.**

Body Surface Area (Clark's BSA) Rule

Estimated child's dose = $\dfrac{\textbf{Child's BSA (m}^2\textbf{) x Adult dose}}{1.73}$

$$BSA\ (m2) = \sqrt{\dfrac{\textbf{height(cm) x weight(kg)}}{3600}}$$

Lamb, TK, Leung, D. More on Simplified Calculation of Body Surface Area. New England Journal of Medicine 1988: 318:1130

Estimation of BSA for Children of "Normal Height and Weight"

Weight		Approximate	Surface Area
kg	lb	Age	(sq m)
3	6.6	Newborn	0.2
6	13.2	3 months	0.3
10	22	1 year	0.45
20	44	5.5 years	0.8
30	66	9 years	1
40	88	12 years	1.3
50	110	14 years	1.5
65	143	Adult	1.7
70	154	Adult	1.76

adapted from West's nomogram

Body Weight Rules

Clark's Rule (patients > 2 yrs)

Child's dose = $\dfrac{\text{Body Wt (lbs) x adult dose}}{150}$

Weight-Based Dosing:

Dose = pediatric dose/kg x child's weight (kg)

Age Rules (less accurate than BSA or weight-based)

Fried's Rule (infants up to 24 mos)

Infant's dose = $\dfrac{\text{age (mos) x adult dose}}{150}$

Young's Rule (2-12 yrs)

Child's dose = $\dfrac{\text{age (yrs) x adult dose}}{\text{age (yrs) + 12}}$

Bronchodilators

Adrenoreceptor Responses

Receptor	Target
alpha-1	Dilates pupils, contracts smooth muscle
beta-1	Stimulates force/rate of heart
beta-2	Bronchodilator of lungs, causes voluntary muscle tremors

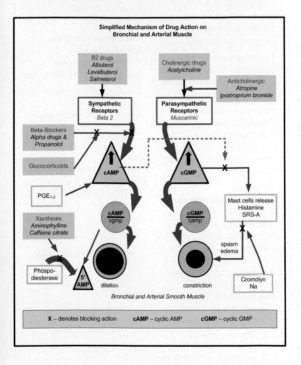

Assessing Response to Bronchodilator Therapy[1]
(AARC CPG)

Indications

Assessment of airflow and other clinical indicators to:

Confirm therapy inappropriateness

Individualized medication dose &/or frequency

Determine patient status during therapy

Determine need for changes in therapy (dose, frequency, types of medication)

Contraindications

Some assessment maneuvers should be postponed during acute, severe distress.

Hazards/Complications

Airway collapse

Bronchoconstriction

Coughing &/or syncope

Inherent hazards of specific procedures

Frequency

Acute, unstable patient –

Pre-therapy: ABGs, full assessment, baseline values

Pre and Post therapy: BS, side effects, vital signs, PEFR, or FEV1 (freq. is based upon acuteness and severity).

Continuous: SpO2

Stable patient-

Hospital: PEF (pre and post therapy initially, then 2 x/ day.

Home: PEF initially 3-4/day than 2x/day, depending on severity of symptoms.

Assessment of Outcome/Monitoring

Pre-therapy (identify):

Clinical indications

Contraindications

Respiratory and CV baseline values

During therapy (identify):

Adverse responses

Clinical changes

Post therapy (identify):

Adverse responses

Therapeutic responses

Lack of therapeutic responses

Trend analysis (identify):

Change in baseline

Need to – change therapy, discontinue therapy, modify dose

Document

Patient responses and progress: BS, lung function (PEFR, FEV, FVC), vital signs, symptoms.

continued next page

Bronchodilator Therapy (continued)

Monitoring	PFT's:
Patient observation:	FEV_1 &/or FVC (improved by 12% increase and 200mL increase) &/or FEF 25-75% improved, ↑PEF.
Accessory muscle use decreased	
General appearance improved	SaO_2, SpO_2 &/or ABG's improved
Sputum expectoration increased	Exercise performance improved
Auscultation:	Ventilator variables improved:
BS improved and volume of air moved is increased	Decreased: auto- PEEP, PIP, Pplat, Raw
Vital signs improved	Increased: expiratory flow
Subjective patient improvement	

1) Adapted from AARC Clinical Practice Guidelines: Assessing Response to Bronchodilator Therapy at Point of Care, *Respiratory Care*, Volume 40, # 12, 1995.

Bronchodilators: Summary of General Side Effects

Pulmonary	Cardiovascular	CNS	Other
Bronchial irritation and edema	↑BP, ↑HR, anginal pain, coronary insufficiency, palpitations, peripheral vasoconstriction	Anxiety, fear, headache, irritability, insomnia, nervousness, restlessness, tremor, vertigo, weakness	Hypersensitivity, reaction to MDI propellants, tachyphylaxis, urinary retention, vomiting, nausea

Anti-Asthma - Mast Cell Stabilizers

Medication	Dosage	Indications/Actions	Contraindications/Notes
cromolyn Na	**INHALED SOLUTION:** 10 mg/mL – 2 mL ampule 2 yr – adult: 20 mg T-Qid **ALLERGEN OR EIA:** Administer single dose 10-15 min, but not > 60 min, before precipitating event.	- Prophylactic maintenance of mild to moderate asthma. - Not for acute exacerbations. - Prevention of allergen or EIA *Prevents release of inflammatory mediators from inflammatory cell types.*	Adverse: Bronchospasm, cough, local irritation, dry mouth, chest tightness, vertigo, unpleasant taste in mouth. Neb solution (may dilute) may be mixed with albuterol.

Anti-asthma - Anti-Leukotrienes

Medication	Dosage	Indications/Actions	
montelukast *Singulair*	**Asthma, seasonal or perennial allergic rhinitis (taken in PM):** 6 mos - 5yrs: 4 mg/day 6 yr - 14 yr: 5 mg/day Adults: 10 mg/day **Bronchoconstriction, EIA (prevention):** Granules: 4 mg/packet Chewable Tablet: 4 mg, 5 mg Tablet: 10 mg	Seasonal/perennial allergic rhinitis, prophylaxis and chronic treatment of asthma, prevention of exercise-induced bronchospasm *Leukotriene receptor antagonist blocks inflammatory mediators*	**Adverse:** Headache, dizziness, dyspepsia, fatigue. May increase liver function test.
zafirlukast *Accolate*	≥ 12 yr: 20 mg Bid 5-11 yr: 10 mg Bid (10, 20 mg tabs)	*Prophylaxis/chronic treatment of asthma*	Same as above Admin 1 hr before or 2 hr after meals.
zileuton *Zyflo*	≥ 12 yr: 600 mg Qid (600 mg tabs) **Immediate Release:** 600 mg; **Extended:** 1,200 mg BID (600 mg tabs)	*Leukotriene inhibitor:* *Prevents formation of inflammatory mediators*	Headache, dizziness, dyspepsia, fatigue, elevated ALT's

12-15

Bronchodilators: Beta Agonists SABA

Medication	Dosage	Indications/Actions	Contraindications/Notes
albuterol *AccuNeb* *ProAir HFA* *Proventil HFA* *Ventolin HFA* *Vospire ER*	See Chart Below	**Bronchoconstriction, Acute and Maintenance** *Stimulates* β1 *(minor),* β2 *(strong)* Onset: 5 min. Peak: 30-60 min Duration: 3-8 hours	Adverse: Slight CV and CNS, hyperglycemia, hypokalemia, tremors May mix with cromolyn or ipratropium neb soln.

ACUTE EXACERBATION (NIH GUIDELINES)

NEBULIZER:
Child: 0.15 mg/kg (minimum 2.5 mg), q 20 min x 3 doses, then 0.15-0.3 mg/kg (up to 10 mg), q 1-4 hrs prn **or** 0.5 mg/kg/hr by continuous neb.
Adult: 2.5-5 mg, q 20 min x 3 doses, then 2.5-10 mg, q 1-4 hrs prn or 10-15 mg/hr by continuous neb.

MDI:
Child: 4-8 puffs, q 20 min x 3 doses, then q 1-4 hrs prn.
Adult: 4-8 puffs, q 20 min for up to 4 hrs, then q 1-4 hrs prn.
MDI (HFA): 90 mcg/puff
Neb. Soln: 5mg/mL (0.5%), 2.5mg/3mL (0.083%), 1.25mg/3mL (0.042%), 0.63mg/3mL (0.021%).
Syrup: 2mg/5mL; Tabs: 2, 4 mg; Extended release tabs: 4, 8 mg

NON-ACUTE (MAINTENANCE)

NEBULIZER:
Child < 12 yrs: 0.15-0.25mg/kg (max 5 mg), q 4-6 hrs prn
Child > 12 yrs – Adult: 2.5 - 5.0 mg, q 4-6 hrs prn

MDI:
Child < 12 yrs: 1-2 puffs qid
Child > 12 yrs – Adult: 2-4 puffs, q 4-6 hrs (max 12 puffs day)

ORAL:
2-6 yrs: 0.1-0.2 mg/kg/dose, tid (max 12 mg/day)
6-12 yrs: 2 mg/dose, T-Qid, extended release 4 mg, Bid (max 24 mg/day)
> 12 yrs – Adults: 2.4 mg/dose, T-Qid, extended release 4-8 mg, Bid (max 32 mg/day)

Bronchodilators: Beta Agonists SABA

Medication	Dosage	Indications/Actions	Contraindications/Notes
lev albuterol *Xopenex* *Xopenex HFA*	**SOLUTION FOR NEBULIZATION:** 0.31 mg/3mL; 0.63 mg/3 mL; 1.25 mg/0.5 mL; 1.25 mg/3 mL **≤ 4 yrs:** 0.31 -1.25 mg, Q4-6 hr, PRN **5-11 yrs:** 0.31 mg Tid (max 0.63 mg Tid) **12 + yrs:** 0.63-1.25 mg, Tid **MDI: 45 mcg/puff** 4+ yrs: 1-2 puffs, Q4-6hr, PRN	**Bronchoconstriction** *R-isomer form of albuterol, stimulates Beta-2 (strong)* **Onset:** 15 min **Peak:** 1.5 hr **Dur:** 5-8 hrs	Slight CV and CNS effects, When using concentrated form (1.25mg/0.5mL), dilution is necessary
pirbuterol acetate *Maxair*	**MDI: 0.2 mg/puff** 12 + yrs: 2 puffs, q 4-6 hr (max: 12 puff/day)	**Bronchoconstriction** *Stimulates β-1 (mild), β-2 (mod)* **Onset:** 5 min **Peak:** ½- 1 hr **Dur:** 3-5 hrs	Same as Above

12-17

Bronchodilators: Beta Agonists LABA

Medication	Dosage	Indications/Actions	Contraindications/ Notes
arformoterol tartrate *Brovana*	**Solution for Nebulization:** 15 mcg / 2 mL **Adults:** 15 mcg BID (do not exceed 30 mcg/day)	**Maintenance treatment of COPD** *Selective long-acting β2-adrenergic receptor agonist*	NOT indicated for acute constriction **SEE INSERT FOR BLACK BOX WARNING**
formoterol fumarate *Foradil* *Performomist*	**Powder/Inhalation:** 12 mcg/capsule (Foradil) **Maintenance Asthma (> 5yr)** Inhale contents of 1 capsule (12 mcg) BID, 12 hrs apart (max 24 mcg/24 hrs) **EIA, prophylaxis (>5 yr)** inhale contents of 1 cap 15 minutes before exercise. Don't repeat within 12 hours **COPD maintenance treatment (Adults)** inhale contents of 1 cap BID (Max 24 mcg/24 hrs)	**Bronchoconstriction** *Long acting selective β2 agonist.* **Onset:** 1-3 min **Peak:** 30-60 min **Duration:** 12 hrs.	Do not use with a spacer. **SEE INSERT FOR BLACK BOX WARNING**

Nebulizer (20 mcg/2 mL) Performomist -- COPD (maintenance) (Adults) 20 mcg BID, max dose 40 mcg/24 hrs

12-18

Bronchodilators: Beta Agonists LABA

salmeterol *Serevent*	**POWDER:** (50 mcg/dose) > 4 yrs: 1 puff, BID, 12 hrs apart max Asthma (>4 yrs; mainten and prevention) COPD (adults) **PREVENTION OF EIA (> 4yrs):** 1 puff (50 mcg) at least 30 minutes prior to exercise. Don't repeat within 12 hrs, and not to be used by patients on salmeterol BID	**Long-Term management of Bronchoconstriction** *Long acting selective β2 agonist.* **Onset:** 10-20 min **Peak:** 3 hrs. **Duration:** 12 hrs.	Not for acute management Diskus not for use with spacer **SEE INSERT FOR BLACK BOX WARNING**
indacaterol *Arcapta Neohaler*	Inhalation capsule: 75 mcg COPD (Adults): inhale 75 mcg once daily	Maintenance treatment of COPD *Long acting selective β2 agonist.* **Onset:** 5 min **Peak:** 1-4 hrs. **Duration:** 24 hrs.	Not for acute management **SEE INSERT FOR BLACK BOX WARNING**

Anti-Cholinergics

Medication	Dosage	Indications/Actions	Contraindications/Notes
aclidinium bromide	**DPI:** 400 μg BID	Maintenance tx of bronchospasm associated with COPD *Long-acting M3 muscarinic antagonist*	Current concerns about administering to patients with underlying cardiovascular disease
ipratropium bromide *Atrovent* *Atrovent HFA*	**Solution for Nebulization:** (0.02%) (500 mcg/2.5 mL) **> 12 yr:** 250-500 mcg, T-Qid **Child:** 250 mcg, Tid **Infant:** 125-250 mcg, Tid **Neonate:** 25 mcg/kg/dose, Tid, max 250 mcg **MDI:** (17 mcg/puff) **< 12 yrs:** 1-2 puffs, Tid (max 6/day) **> 12 yr:** 2-3 puffs, Qid (max 12/day)	Treatment of bronchospasm associated with COPD, bronchitis/emphysema *Anticholinergic: blocks acetyl-choline + potentiates β2 stim.* **ACUTE EXACERBATION:** **> 12 yrs:** 500 mcg, q 20 min x 3 doses, then q 2-4 hrs. **< 12 yrs:** 250 mcg, q 20 min x 3 doses, then q 2-4 hrs. **MDI:** (all ages) (NIH Guidelines): 4-8 puffs, q 20 minutes as needed for up to 3 hrs	**Adverse:** mucus viscosity, local inflammation, dry mouth, pupil dilation May mix with Albuterol (See page 12-34) **Not to be used as a rescue inhaler**

Medication	Dosage	Indications/Actions	Contraindications/Doses
tiotropium bromide *Spiriva (HandiHaler)*	**DPI: 18 mcg** 1 inhalation/day	Maintenance tx of COPD Action same as Atrovent **Onset:** 30 min **Peak:** 3 hrs **Duration:** >24 hrs	**Adverse:** dry mouth, urinary retention, constipation, increased HR, blurred vision, glaucoma Not to be used as a rescue inhaler

Xanthines

Medication	Dosage	Indications/Actions	Contraindications/Doses
aminophylline	**NEONATAL APNEA:** Load: 5 mg/kg over 30" (IV or PO) Maintenance: 5 mg/kg/day, q 12 hrs **BRONCHODILATION:** Load: 6 mg/kg over 20-30 min (IV) Maintenance: **Neonate:** 0.2mg/kg/hr; **6 wk – 6 mo:** 0.5mg/kg/hr **6mo – 12mo:** 0.6-0.7 mg/kg/hr	**Bronchoconstriction** **Neonatal apnea** **Bronchodilation** **(inhibits phospho-di-esterase)** *Stimulates rate and depth of respiration, pulmonary vasodilation* **1-9 yrs:** 1-1.2 mg/kg/hr **9-12 yrs:** 0.9 mg/kg/hr (+ young smokers) **> 12 yrs:** 0.7 mg/kg/hr (+ older nonsmokers)	↑CV and CNS effects, many systemic effects Toxicity > 20 mg/L (> 15 mg/L in neonates)

Alpha-1 Antitrypsin Disorder

Medication	Dosage	Indications/Actions	Contraindications/Notes
Alpha 1 Proteinase Inhibitor *Human*	60 mg/kg once weekly For IV use only, infuse over 30 min. **POWDER FOR RECONSTITUTION:** **Aralast NP:** 500 mg, 1000 mg vials **Prolastin:** 1000 mg vial **Zemaira:** 1000 mg vial **Glassia:** 1000 mg (50 mL) Injection solution	**Congenital alpha 1- antitrypsin deficiency.** *Replaces enzymes lost in patients with this disorder*	Hypersensitivity and anaphylactic reactions **Adverse:** ↑ALT, AST, Headache, Musculoskeletal discomfort, pharyngitis, allergic reactions, fever, light headedness

12-22

Medication	Dosage	Indications/Actions	
aztreonam *Cayston*	**Powder for Reconstitution:** Oral inhalation (75 mg) ≥ 7 yrs: 75 mg Tid for 28 days Do not repeat for 28 days after completion	Management of *P. aeruginosa* infection in cystic fibrosis	Administer bronchodilator first Administer alone (do not mix with other nebulized meds) Watch for bronchospasm
colistimethate Na *Coly-Mycin*	**Solution for Nebulization:** 75mg/mL 50-75 mg every 8-12 hours	Management of P. aeruginosa *Antibiotic for G-activity (pseudomonal activity)*	Dilute dose in NS to 4 mL Administer via Pari LC plus nebulizer & filter valve set Mix immediately before admir.

12-23

Anti-Infectives

Medication	Dosage	Indications/Actions	Contraindications/Notes
pentamidine isethionate *NebuPent*	**- 5+ yrs:** 300 mg (1 vial), q 3-4 wks **- <5 yrs:** 8 mg/kg/dose (up to 300mg) - Deliver via Respirgard II neb at 5-7 LPM at 50 PSI until gone	**Prophylaxis of Pneumocystis pneumonia** *Anti-protozoan*	Do not mix with other drugs Mix 300 mg (1 vial) w/ 6mL sterile water Administer bronchodilator prior to tx Adverse Reactions: Irritation, cough, fatigue, SOB, bronchospasm, metallic taste, systemic effects
Note: Caregiver precautions – administer only in an isolated room with separate air circulating system and neg. pressure. Minimize environmental drug exposure. Wear gown, gloves, mask and goggles. Nebulize to <3 μm MMAD.			
ribavirin *Virazole*	**AEROSOL:** 2 grams over 2 hrs 3x/day (60 mg/mL - 6 grams reconstituted w/ 100 mL of sterile, preservative-free water, for 3-7 days.	**Severe lower respiratory tract infection (bronchiolitis, viral pneumonia)** *Antiviral (RSV/influenza A & B)*	Not recommended for intubated patients Do not mix with other drugs Deliver with SPAG-2
May cause adverse effects in healthcare workers (especially for pregnant women). Use of neg. pressure room, scavenging devices, and resp. masks is recommended.		Watch for acute respiratory deterioration + CV effects. Deliver aerosol into mask or hood, (not ET tube and/or vent).	

Medication	Dosage	Indications/Actions	
tobramycin *Tobi*	**AEROSOL:** *> 6 yr:* 300 mg, q 12 hr (300 mg/5 mL), repeat in cycles of 28 days on, 28 days off. *<6yr:* 100 mg, q 12h	**Management of P. aeruginosa infections in cystic fibrosis patients.** *Antibiotic for G- activity (Pseudomonal activity)*	Don't dilute/mix w/ other drugs. Admin via Pari®LC plus nebulizer + filter valve set Adverse Reactions: multiple (review mfr insert)
zanamivir *Relenza*	POWDER/INHALATION: 5 mg/blister influenza treatment: ≥ 7 yrs: 10 mg inhaled Bid influenza prophylaxis: ≥ 5 yrs: 10 mg inhaled, 1/day × 10 days	*Treatment of influenza A or B*	Use a dischaler Not recommended for use in patients with airway disease

Cystic Fibrosis Transmembrane Conductance Regulator (CFTR) Potentiator

Medication	Dosage	Indications/Actions	Contraindications/Notes
Ivacaftor *Kalydeco*	One 150mg tablet, q 12 hours	*Indicated for the treatment of cystic fibrosis (CF) in patients age 6 years and older who have a G551D mutation in the CFTR gene.* *A cystic fibrosis transmembrane conductance regulator (CFTR) potentiator*	Adverse: URI, headache, stomach ache, rash, diarrhea, and dizziness. It is not effective in CF patients with two copies of the F508 mutation in the CFTR gene, which is the most common mutation that results in CF. If a patient's mutation status is not known, an FDA-cleared CF mutation test should be used to determine whether the G551D mutation is present.

IgE Blockers

Medication	Dosage	Indications/Actions	Complications/Notes
omalizumab *Xolair*	**>12 yrs:** 150 - 375 mg, subcutaneous q. 2-4 weeks (varies according to Ige level/wgt)	**Mod-Sev persistent asthma /inadeq. control w/ steroids** *Humanized IgG1 monoclonal antibody*	Bruising, erythema See **Black Box Warning** for this medication

Mucoactives

Medication	Dosage			Indications/Actions	Complications/Notes
acetylcysteine *Mucomyst*	**INHALATION SOLUTION:** T-Qid			**Tenacious mucous** *Breaks mucus disulfide bonds.* *Decreases mucous viscosity.* **Peak:** 5-10 min **Duration:** > 1 hr	**Adverse:** Bronchospasm (administer bronchodilator before use), stomatitis, nausea, rhinitis, unpleasant odor/taste. Overmobilization of secretions
	Age	**10%**	**20%**		
	> 12 yr:	10 mL	5 mL		
	Child:	6-10 mL	3-5 mL		
	Infant:	2-4 mL	1-2 mL		
	20% is diluted 1:1 with H2O or NS				
	INSTILLATION: q 1-4 hrs, prn 1-2 mL (20%) (200 mg/mL) (100 mg/mL) 2-4 mL (10%) (100 mg/mL)				
dornase alfa-dnase *Pulmozyme*	**INHALATION SOLUTION:** 3 mos-adult: 2.5 mg, 1-2 x/day (1 mg/mL, 2.5 mL amp)			**Tenacious mucus (decreases infection)** *Dornase alpha recombinant, decrease viscocity*	Same as acetylcysteine -- Do not mix or dilute with other drugs.

12-27

Inhaled Analgesics

Medication	Dosage	Indications/Actions	Contraindications/Notes
Lidocaine *(off-label)*	Nebulized- 2-4ml of 1%-4% lidocaine. Dosing varies greatly in literature. (Start with lower dosing)	Pre-bronchoscopy. Pre-nasogastric tube insertion. Intractable cough. Has also been used to treat asthma. Inhibits Na ion channels.	Use with caution. May cause airway irritation, reduced gag reflex leading to aspiration.
Morphine Sulfate *(off-label)*	Nebulized- Starting dose- 2-5mg Q4prn Mix with 3ml normal saline. BAN recommended. (Higher doses and escalating frequency may be needed).	Dyspnea, pain and cough in palliative care patients. Binds to opioid receptors, producing analgesia (opioid agonist).	Use with caution. May cause bronchospasm, respiratory depression, constipation and nausea. May pre-treat with a bronchodilator or have bronchodilator ready. Escalating doses with more frequent treatments may be necessary. Nebulize as an alternate route of delivery other than PO or IV.

12-28

Inhaled Epinephrine

Medication	Dosage	Indications/Actions	Contraindications/Notes

Racemic epinephrine
S2
Primatene
	INHALATION SOLUTION:
	22.5 mg/mL (0.5 mL)
	(2.25%)
	0.25-0.5 mL (2.25%) in 2.5 mL diluent
	
	CROUP:
	< 5 kg: 0.25 mL/dose; > 5 kg: 0.5 mL/dose
	
	S2: 1-3 inhalations, q 3 hrs, PRN
	  Do not administer more frequently than q 2 hrs
	Primatene (OTC) Inhaler:
	≥ 4 yrs
	  1 inhalation, wait 1 minute, may use once more
	  Do not use again for at least 3 hrs
		Bronchoconstriction
		Tracheobronchial inflammation (post extubation, etc.)
		Nasal congestion
		
		Stimulates:
		  alpha-1 (mild)
		  beta-1 (medium)
		  beta-2 (mild)
		Duration: ½-2 hrs
			Milder effects than epinephrine
			Rebound airway edema, cardiac arrhythmias, chest pain, trembling, dizziness, headache
			Use min # doses to get response

Phosphodiesterase Inhibitors

Medication	Dosage	Indications/Actions	Contraindications/Notes
roflumilast *Daliresp*	Adults: 500 mcg PO Once Daily 500 mcg tabs	COPD prophylaxis (reduction in acute exacerbations) Recommended for severe or very severe COPD w/ bronchitic component PDE4 Inhibitor (may affect enzyme that contributes to bronchoconstriction and inflammation)	DO NOT use as a bronchodilator Should not be used for relief of acute bronchospasm Contraindicated in pts with liver impairment, not recommended in tandem with rifampin, carbamezepine, phenytoin, phenobarbital.

Pulmonary Vasodilators

Medication	Dosage	Indications/Actions	Contraindications/Notes
iloprost *Ventavis*	INHALATION SOLUTION: 10 mcg/mL; 20 mcg/mL Initial: 2.5 mcg inhaled, ↑dose to 5 mcg, 6-9 x/day No more than q 2 hr during waking hrs Max/day: 45 mcg	Pulmonary hypertensive arterial disease	Use I-Neb or Prodose AAD System
Other Pulmonary Vasodilators:	ambrisentan (Letairis) - tab bosentan (Tracleer) - tab	epoprostenol (Flolan, Veletri) - IV sildenafil (Revatio) - tab	tadalafil (Adcirca) - tab treprostinil (Tyvaso, Remodulin) – inhal/inject

5 A's of Smoking

ASK	every patient should be asked if they use tobacco every time you see them
ADVISE	non-judgmentally, advise all smokers to quit
ASSESS	assess the smoker for motivation (are they ready to quit?)
ASSIST	develop a plan with the smoker to quit, discuss pharmacological options, recommend counseling, provide adequate materials
ARRANGE	directly follow-up on regular intervals, or arrange for adequate follow-up

Fagerstrom Test for Nicotine Dependence

How soon after you wake up do you smoke your first cigarette?	5 min or less	*3 points*
	6-30 minutes	*2 points*
	31-60 minutes	*1 point*
	60+ minutes	*0 points*
Do you find it hard to refrain from smoking in places where it is forbidden?	Yes	*1 point*
	No	*0 points*
What cigarette would you hate most to give up?	First Morning	*1 point*
	Any other	*0 point*
How many cigarettes per day do you smoke?	10 or less	*0 points*
	11-20	*1 point*
	21-30	*2 points*
	31 or more	*3 points*
Do you smoke more during the first hours after waking?	Yes	*1 point*
	No	*0 points*
Do you smoke if you are so ill you can't get out of bed?	Yes	*1 point*
	No	*0 points*

≥ 6 indicates a high level of dependence

Smoking Cessation

Medication	Dosage	Summary of Action	Contraindications/Notes
varenicline *Chantix*	**Start Chantix 1 week prior to quit date.** -1mg BID following a 1 week titration: Days 1-3: 0.5mg qd Days 4-7: 0.5mg bid Day 8+: 1mg bid 12 wk course of treatment, then another 12 weeks if success during 1st course	*Binds with neuronal nicotinic acetylcholine receptors. Produces agonist activity (blocks the reward/reinforcement a person may feel as a result of smoking).*	**Side Effects may be common:** -serious neuropsychiatric symptoms, including changes in behavior, agitation, depressed mood, suicidal ideation and suicidal behavior nausea (mild-moderate, persistent), sleep disturbance, flatulence, constipation.
bupropion *Zyban*	**Tablets (150 mg)** Start 2wks before quitting 150 mg/day x 3 days *then* 150mg BID for 7-12 weeks	*Unknown, may have nonadrenergic or dopaminic effects (decreases some of the cravings for cigarettes)*	Should not be taken with MAO Inhibitors, or people with seizure disorders. **See insert for Black Box Warning**
Nasal Spray *Nicotrol NS*	Nasal Spray (0.5mg nicotine per spray) 1-2 doses per hour, not to exceed 40mg (80 sprays) per day	*Nicotine Replacement therapies decrease withdrawal symptoms by giving measured, smaller doses of nicotine*	Patient should be instructed to not smoke concurrently Use should not exceed 6 mos.

12-32

Smoking Cessation

Medication	Dosage	Summary of Action	Contraindications/Notes
		Nicotine Replacement therapies decrease withdrawal symptoms by giving measured, smaller doses of nicotine	
Transdermal patch *Nicotrol*	**15 mg/patch for 6 weeks** >10 cigarettes/day: Apply 1 patch in the A.M.; remove before bed (don't wear overnight)		**Adverse:** skin irritation, insomnia **Precautions:** pregnancy, heart disease
Transdermal Patch *Nicoderm CQ*	**Patch 7, 14, 21 mg/ patch** **<10 cig/day:** 14mg for 16-24hr x 6wk *then* 7mg for 16-24hr x 2 wk **>10 cig/day:** 21mg for 16-24hr x 6wk *then* 14mg for 16-24hr x 2 wk *then* 7mg for 16-24hr x 2 wk		
Gum/ Lozenges *Nicorette Gum,* *Commit* *Lozenge*	**Gum:** 2, 4 mg (max: 30 pcs/day) **Lozenges:** 2, 4 mg (max: 20 loz/day) 2-4 mg over 30 min q 1-2 hr x 6wk, *then* q. 2-4 hr x 3 wk, *then* q. 4-8 hr x 3 wk		Dentures Pregnancy Heart Disease
Oral Inhaler *Nicotrol*	10mg cartridges, 4mg delivered 6-16 cartridges per day Patient should be instructed in controlling depth and frequency of inhalation		**Adverse:** dyspepsia, cough, mouth irritation/burning Avoid in COPD, asthma, pregnancy and heart disease

Steroids

Medication	Dosage	Summary of Action	Contraindications/Notes
beclomethasone (QVAR) budesonide (Pulmicort, Flexhaler Pulmicort Respules) fluticasone (Flovent) mometasone furoate (Asmanex) ciclesonide (Alvesco)	See insert for dosing information	*Anti-inflammatory for maintenance with prophylactic treatment of asthma*	Cough, sneezing, dysphonia, pharyngitis, voice alteration, headache, dyspepsia, nasal congestion, and oral candidiasis. Rinsing the mouth with water after use will help minimize dry mouth, hoarseness, and oral candidiasis.

Wetting Agents

Medication	Dosage	Indications/Actions	Contraindications/Notes
water sterile, distilled	Intermittent or continuous nebulization	**Thick Secretions** *Humidify/thin/liquefy secretions*	Potential mucosal irritation, over-hydration, bronchospasm
Saline: Hypotonic (0.45% NaCl)		*Diluent of drugs*	Same as above Less irritating than H2O
Saline: Isotonic (0.9%)			Bronchospasm
Saline: Hypertonic	**Aerosol:** intermittent only (2-5 mL)	**Sputum Induction** *Above + osmotic transudat.*	Bronchospasm, mucosal irritation, edema, ↑ blood Na⁺

Combination: Corticosteroid and LABA

Medication	Dosage	Summary of Action	
budesonide and formoterol *Symbicort*	Inhalation ≥ 5 yrs 80mcg b.udesonide/ 4.5 formoterol 2 inhalations BID Inhalation: 160 mcg budesonide/ 4.5 mcg formoterol 2 inhalations BID	Long-term maintenance treatment of asthma in persons over 12 years old, who are not easily controlled with corticosteroid and occassional use of a SABA. *Combines action of systemic corticosteroid and LABA*	SEE BLACK BOX WARNING SYMBICORT: Instruct patients to shake inhaler for a full 5 seconds prior to using, to mix medications. Rinse mouth after use Adverse: sore nose/throat, headache, stomach irritation, sinusitis, cardiovascular side effects
fluticasone and salmeterol *Advair*	DPI: 100/50, 250/50, 500/50 (fluticasone/salmeterol) Asthma (100/50, 250/50) COPD (250/50) 1 inhalation BID, max 2/day HFA (LT maint.): (45/21, 115/21, 230/21) >12 yrs: 2 inh. BID, max 4/day	LT maintenance treatment of asthma in persons > 12 yrs Maintenance treatment (250/50)of airway obstruction associated with Chronic Bronchitis	Contraindicated as a rescue inhaler
See insert for recommended dosages for Asthma pts not adequately controlled by corticosteroids			

Combination: Corticosteroid and LABA

Medication	Dosage	Summary of Action	Contraindications/Notes
mometa-sone and formoterol	INHALATION 100 mcg/5 mcg 200 mcg/5 mcg ≥ 12 yrs: 2 inhalations, Bid Max 4 inhalations/day	Long term maintenance treatment of asthma	SEE BLACK BOX WARNING
Dulera			Same as Above

Combination: Anti-Cholinergic and SABA

Medication	Dosage	Indications/Actions	Contraindications/Notes
ipratropium bromide and albuterol *Duoneb*	AEROSOL (0.5 mg ipratropium/2.5 mg albuterol) 3 mL nebulized QID, with 2 additional doses if needed	COPD with bronchospasm *SABA and anticholinergic combined effects, which are thought to have a greater effect than either drug independently*	Do not administered with sym-pathomimetics/MAO inhibitors Paradoxical Bronchospasm
ipratropium bromide and albuterol sulfate	MDI: 18 mcg ipratropium bromide and 103 mcg albuterol sulfate		Caution with glaucoma, prostatic hypertrophy
Combivent	2 inhalations QID, not to exceed 12 inhalations a day		

12-36

Medications Affecting Ventilation

Drugs that Cause Respiratory Depression

Ethyl alcohol

Hallucinogens (PCP, angel dust)

Narcotics: codeine, heroin, propoxyphene (Darvon), oxycodone (Percodan), fentanyl (Sublimaze), hydromorphone (Dialaudid), meperidine (Demerol), morphine

Sedatives/Hypnotics:

chloral hydrate, diazepam (Valium), lorazepam (Ativan), midazolan (Versed), zolpidem (Ambien)

Barbiturates:

phenobarbital, pentobarbital, thiopental (Pentothal)

Anesthetics: Propofol (Diprivan)

Paralytics (should not be administered without appropriate sedation, pt will cease ventilatory effort, airway must be managed). Several popular drugs, some of which have reversal agents (notable exception: succinylchonine, or "succs")

Drugs that Cause Respiratory Stimulation

Acids (CO2, HCl, NH3Cl)

Adrenergic agents: ampheamine, ephedrine, norepinephrine

Alcohol: ethylene glycol (antifreeze)

Analeptics: doxapram (Dopram)

Benzodiazepine antagonists: flumazenil (Romazicon)

Diuretics: carbonic anhydrase inhibitors: acetazolamide

Hormones: ACTH, estrogen, insulin, progesterone, thyroxine

Irritants: ammonia, ether

Narcotic antagonist: naloxone (Narcan)

Salicylates: aspirin

Xanthines: aminophylline, caffeine, theophylline

See Oakes' Ventilator Management for detailed information on Critical Care Drugs, inlcuding Diuretics, Anticoagulants, Paralytics and Paralytic-Reversal Drugs

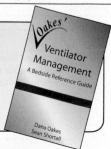

Oakes'

Ventilator Management
A Bedside Reference Guide

Dana Oakes
Sean Shortall

Common Cardiovascular Drugs

Anti-Arrhythmics

adenosine (Adenocard)
amiodarone
diltiazem (Cardizem)
disopyramide
doletilide
esmolol
fosphenytoin (Cerebyx)
ibutilide (Corvert)
lidocaine (Xylocaine)

mexiletine
phenytoin (Dilantin)
procainamide
  (Procan, Pronestyl)
propafenone (Rhythmol)
propranolol (Inderal)
quinidine (Cardoquin)
tocainide (Tonocard)
verapamil (Calan, Isoptin)

Vasodilators (Vessel Dilation)

captopril (Capoten)
enalapril (Vasotec)
fenoldopam (Corlopam)
isoproterenol (Isuprel)
hydralazine (Apresoline)
labetalol (Nomodyne, Trandate)
nesiritide

nicardipine (Cardene)
nitroglycerin
phentolamine (Regitime)
sodium nitroprusside
  (Nipride, Nitropress)
tolazoline (Priscoline)

Inotropics (↑ Cardiac Contractility)

amrinone (Inocor)
digoxin (Lanoxin)
dobutamine (Dobutrex)
dopamine (Intropin)

epinephrine (Adrenalin)
isoproterenol (Isuprel)
milrinone (Primacor)

Vasopressors (Vessel Constriction)

ephedrine (Bofedrol, Ephed)
metaraminol bitartate
  (Aramine)

norepinephrine or levartere-
  nol (Levophed)
phenylephrine (Neosynephrine)

See Oakes' Hemodynamic
Monitoring for expanded in-
formation on Cardiovascular
Physiology

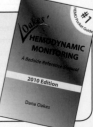

13 Resuscitation (BLS/ACLS)

!

This Chapter is a Summary of the *2010 American Heart Association* Guidelines for Cardiopulmonary Resuscitation and Emergency Cardiovascular Care Science

CPR

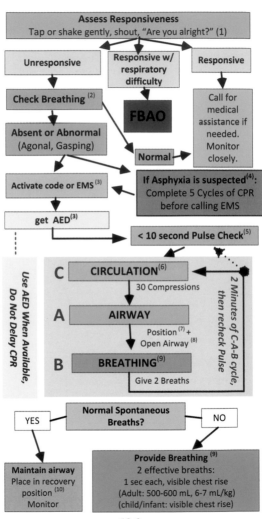

Assess Responsiveness
Tap or shake gently, shout, "Are you alright?" (1)

Unresponsive	Responsive w/ respiratory difficulty	Responsive

Check Breathing [2]

Absent or Abnormal
(Agonal, Gasping)

FBAO

Call for medical assistance if needed. Monitor closely.

Normal

Activate code or EMS [3]

If Asphyxia is suspected [4]:
Complete 5 Cycles of CPR before calling EMS

get AED [3]

< 10 second Pulse Check [5]

Use AED When Available, Do Not Delay CPR

C   **CIRCULATION** [6]

30 Compressions

A   **AIRWAY**

Position [7] + Open Airway [8]

B   **BREATHING** [9]

Give 2 Breaths

2 Minutes of C-A-B cycle, then recheck Pulse

Normal Spontaneous Breaths?

YES   NO

Maintain airway
Place in recovery position [10]
Monitor

Provide Breathing [9]
2 effective breaths:
1 sec each, visible chest rise
(Adult: 500-600 mL, 6-7 mL/kg)
(child/infant: visible chest rise)

CPR

Assess Signs of Circulation [10]

≤ 10 sec { Check for coughing, breathing, movement
{ Check pulse: Adult + Child: carotid or femoral; < 1yr: brachial

Definite Pulse (confident)
Ventilate as needed
1 sec each
Visible chest rise
Adult: 10-12/min (q. 5-6 sec)
Child/Infant: 12-20/min (q 3-5 sec)

Activate EMS (if not already)
Reassess pulse q. 2 mins (≤ 10 sec)

No Pulse (or not confident)
or
Child/Infant w/ HR<60 + poor perfusion

Provide Chest Compressions [11]

Early AED Use

		Infant (< 1yr)	Child (1yr-puberty)	Adult
Push Hard - Push Fast - Allow full recoil	Technique	2 fingers (1 rescuer) 2 thumb-encircling hands (2 rescuers)	1 or 2 hands	2 hands
	Place	Just below nipple line	At nipple line (center of chest)	
	Depth	at least 1/3 depth of chest (1.5 in for infant, 2 in for child)		at least 2 inches (5 cm)
	Rate	At Least 100/minute		
	Ratio	*Unsecured airway* 30/2 : 1 rescuer 15/2 : 2 rescuers		*Unsecured airway* 30/2 : 1 or 2 rescuers
		Secured airway & 2 rescuers 8-10 breaths/min (q 6-8 sec) (No pause or synchronization for breaths)		

Peform 5 cycles (approx 2 min) [12]
(minimize interruptions)

Then
Reassess breathing + circulation (take ≤ 10 sec)
Continue CPR + Reasses q. 2 min (5 cycles)

13-3

FOOTNOTES

(1) Assess for Safety and Response - First ensure scene is safe. Suspected head or neck injury: do not shake; move only if necessary.

(2) Assess Breathing - While assessing for response, quickly distinguish adequate from inadequate (weak or agonal [reflex gasping]) breathing.

(3) Activate Code (or EMS) and get AED
> 1 Rescuer - Activate code, get AED (If readily available; use as appropriate (See AED section), then begin CPR
> 2 Rescuers - One rescuer begins CPR, while the other activates the code (or EMS) and retrieves an AED (if available).

AED -
- Shockable rhythm (child and adult only)
- Give 1 shock, immediately resume CPR (beginning with compressions), do not check pulse.
- After 5 cycles, analyze rhythm, deliver another shock if indicated.

> **Infants** (< 1 yr) - For infants (<1 year of age), a manual defibrillator is preferred. If a manual defibrillator is not available, an AED with pediatric dose attenuation is desirable. If neither is available, an AED without a dose attenuator may be used
> **Children** - 2 Joules/kg first attempt; at least 4 J/kg subsequent attempt not to exceed 10 J/kg or the adult maximum dose.
> **Ages 1- 8 yrs** - use pediatric dose-attenuator system, if available (See AED section)

(4) Current guidelines recommend differentiating between Cardiac Arrest (Sudden Collapse) and Suspected Asphyxia (such as drowning). For Suspected/Presumed asphyxia, the priority is CPR: therefore provide chest compressions with rescue breathing for 5 cycles (2 minutes) before calling EMS.

(5) Check Pulse - Take no less than 5, but no more than 10 sec
> Adult/child: use carotid or femoral
> Infant < 1 yr: use brachial

If no pulse (or not confident) or child/infant < 60/min and poor perfusion: provide chest **compressions**

> **If definite pulse:** ventilate as needed ventilation rates are rescue breaths only, NOT CPR RATES
> **Adult:** 10-12/min (q 5-6 sec)
> **Child/Infant:** 12-20/min (q 3-5 sec)

(6) **Chest Compressions** - Equal compression/relaxation ratio. Allow
   chest to return to normal position without lifting hands from chest.
   Reason: allows for refilling of heart chambers with blood.

2 Rescuers:
   Unsecured airway - Pause compressions for ventilations. Begin com-
      pressions at peak inspiration of 2nd breath.
   Secured airway - Do not pause or synchronize for ventilations.

   Note: Do not monitor and/or gauge chest compression force as
      adequate by palpable carotid or femoral pulse (may be venous).

   Two rescuers should change compressor/ventilator roles approxi-
      mately every 2 minutes (5 cycles) to prevent tiring (increases risk of
      ineffective compressions)

(7) **Position** -
   Victim: supine, arms alongside on firm, flat surface.   Move head,
   shoulders, and torso as one unit without twisting.

   Rescuer: kneeling beside victim's thorax (Fig 13).

(8) **Open Airway** -
   Head tilt - chin lift: preferred when no evidence of head or neck
      trauma (Fig 1).
   Jaw thrust: use when suspect cervical spine injury. Do not tilt head
      back or sideways (Fig 2). Use spinal motion restriction rather than
      immobilization devices. Note: if jaw thrust does not open the
      airway: use head tilt - chin lift.
   Open mouth and remove any visible foreign material, vomitus, or
   loose dentures (Fig 20). A blind finger sweep is no longer recommended because of the risk of pushing a foreign body further into
   the airway.

(9) **Provide Breathing** - Avoid large, rapid or forceful breaths. Do not
   deliver more volume or force than is needed to produce visible chest
   rise. Use mouth to mouth/nose for infants (See ACLS Section)

(10) **Recovery Position** -
   Unresponsive victims with normal breathing and effective circula-
      tion. Place victim as near as possible to a true and stable lateral
      position (lower arm in front of body) with head dependent, no
      pressure on chest, and good observation/access to airway (Fig 3).
   Suspected spinal injury: move to recovery position only if open
      airway cannot be maintained (eg., lone rescuer must leave victim
      to get help). May opt for lower arm above head, with head on arm
      and knees bent.

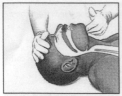

Fig. 1. Head tilt-chin lift

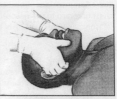

Fig. 2. Jaw thrust
(without head tilt)

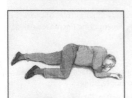

Fig. 3. Recovery position

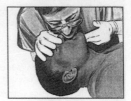

Fig. 4. Mouth-to-mouth
rescue breathing

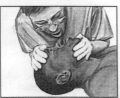

Fig. 5. Mouth-to-nose
rescue breathing

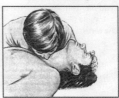

Fig. 6. Mouth-to-stoma
rescue breathing

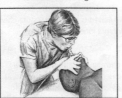

Fig. 7. Mouth-to-mask
cephalic technique

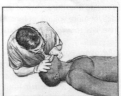

Fig. 8. Mouth-to-mask
lateral technique

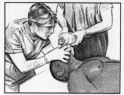

Fig. 9. Two rescuer use
of the bag mask

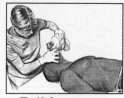

Fig. 10. One rescuer use
of the bag mask

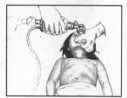

Fig. 11. Bag-mask ventilation for child victim
A, 1 rescuer; B, 2 rescuers

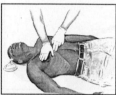

Fig. 12. Positioning of rescuer's
hands for chest compressions

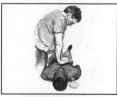

Fig. 13. Position of rescuer
for chest compressions

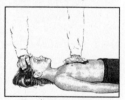

Fig. 14. One hand chest
compression in child

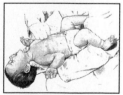

Fig. 15. One rescuer
infant CPR while carrying

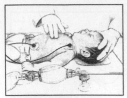

Fig. 16. Two finger
chest compression

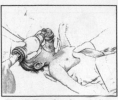

Fig. 17. Two thumb-encircling
hands chest compression

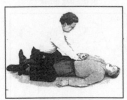

Fig. 18. Heimlich maneuver
in unresponsive victim

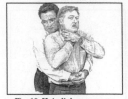

Fig. 19. Heimlich maneuver,
victim standing

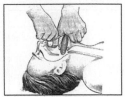

Fig. 20. Finger sweep

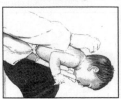

Fig. 21. Infant back blows

FBAO - FOREIGN BODY AIRWAY OBSTRUCTION

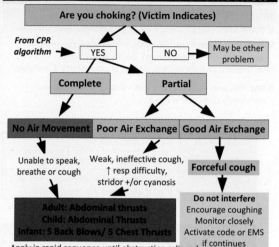

Are you choking? (Victim Indicates)

From CPR algorithm → | YES | | NO | → May be other problem

Complete | **Partial**

No Air Movement | **Poor Air Exchange** | **Good Air Exchange**

Unable to speak, breathe or cough | Weak, ineffective cough, ↑ resp difficulty, stridor +/or cyanosis | **Forceful cough**

Adult: Abdominal thrusts
Child: Abdominal Thrusts
Infant: 5 Back Blows/ 5 Chest Thrusts

Apply in rapid sequence until obstruction relieved
In adult or child: if not effective, consider chest thrusts

Do not interfere
Encourage coughing
Monitor closely
Activate code or EMS if continues

Victim Becomes Unconscious
Lower victim to ground (supine)
Activate code or EMS

Begin CPR
Go to BLS - Airway

Look into mouth before giving breaths – finger sweep ONLY if you see solid material

Notes:

Infant/child –

5 Back blows/5 Chest thrusts: one every sec as needed, same location and technique as chest compressions

Abdominal thrusts not recommended for infants (<1 yr)

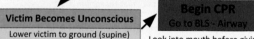

Sudden respiratory distress (coughing, gagging, and/or stridor) unaccompanied by fever, congestion, hoarseness, drooling or lethargy are indicative of infections such as epiglottitis or croup. The child must be taken immediately to an emergency facility because back blows or chest thrusts will not relieve the obstruction.

Late pregnancy – use chest thrusts

Obesity – use chest thrusts (if rescuer cannot encircle abdomen)

13-9

AED - AUTOMATED EXTERNAL DEFIBRILLATOR

Witnessed Arrest	Unwitnessed Arrest
Use AED ASAP	Give 5 cycles CPR (2 min), then use AED

Shockable rhythm: Give one shock, immediately resume CPR (beginning with compressions), do not check pulse.
After 5 cycles, analyze rhythm, deliver another shock if indicated.

Notes: Rescuers must practice minimizing the time between compressions to give a shock.

Infants (< 1 yr) –

1st Preference:	Manual Defibrillator
2nd Preference:	AED with pediatric dose attenuator
3rd Preference	AED without a dose attenuator may be used if above two are not available

Children –

1st Attempt	2 Joules/kg
Subsequent Attempts	at least 4 Joules/kg, *not to exceed 10 Joules/kg* *or the adult maximum dose*

Ages 1- 8 yrs – use pediatric dose-attenuator system, if available.

Airway

Adjuncts

Oropharyngeal Airway	• Use only in unconscious (unresponsive) patients with no cough or gag reflex. • Should be inserted only by trained personnel. • Note: Incorrect insertion can displace the tongue into hypopharynx.
Nasopharyngeal Airway	• Useful in patients with (or at risk of developing) airway obstruction (particularly clenched jaw). • May be better tolerated than oropharyngeal in patients not deeply unconscious. • Caution in patients with severe cranial facial injury. • May be easily obstructed by secretions in infants

Advanced Airways (General)	
Advantages	• Isolation of airway • Reduced risk of aspiration • Potentially improved ventilation and oxygenation • Allows CPR without interruption of compressions • Ability to use capnography to monitor quality of CPR, optimize chest compressions, and detect ROSC during chest compressions
Disadvantages	• Insertion may require interruption of chest compressions. • May defer insertion until patient fails to respond to initial CPR or demonstrates ROSC. • Risk of unrecognized esophageal intubation
Notes	• Optimal method (bag-mask, ET tube, Combitube, or LMA) depends on rescuer experience, patient's condition, and system. • Healthcare providers must maintain knowledge and skills through frequent practice with these devices. • Once advanced airway is in place, 2 rescuers no longer deliver cycles of CPR. • Infants and children: In out-of-hospital setting, bag and mask ventilation preferred over intubation, if transport is short.

Endotracheal (ET) Tube	
Indications	• Inability to ventilate unconscious patient with bag and mask • Absence of airway protective reflexes (coma, cardiac arrest)
Advantages	• Patent airway • Drug administration • High Oxygen delivery route • Specific VT delivery • Cuff protection • Permits suctioning
Technique	• Inserter must be trained and experienced. • Minimize the number and duration of interruptions to chest compressions (be fully prepared to insert when compressing rescuer pauses) to < 10 seconds. Compressions should resume as soon as the tube passes through the vocal cords. Provide adequate ventilation/compressions between attempts. • Pulse oximetry and ECG should be monitored continuously during intubation of patient with a perfusing rhythm. Interrupt attempt if oxygenation/ventilation is needed.
Verify Placement	• Auscultation: BS equal/bilateral, BS absent over epigastrum • Chest expansion • ETCO$_2$ detector or EDD (see 10-24) • Continuous waveform capnography is recommended • SpO$_2$ only if a perfusing rhythm
Notes	• No one single confirmation technique is completely reliable (including H$_2$O vapor). If any doubt: Use laryngoscope to visualize tube passing through vocal cords. If still doubt, remove tube. • Remove tube at once if hear stomach gurgling and see no chest expansion. • Children: Body Length is most reliable (use tape), but **in emergency use:** |		
	3.5 mm ID	3.0 mm ID
	4.0 mm ID	3.5 mm ID
	3.5 + (age/4)	3.5 + (age/4)	

Notes	• If an intubated pt's condition deteriorates, consider the following (DOPE): • **D**isplacement of the tube • **O**bstruction of the tube • **P**neumothorax • **E**quipment failure
Alternatives	• Laryngeal Mask Airway (LMA). May be advantageous when access to pt is limited, presence of unstable neck injury, or positioning for intubation impossible • Esophageal-tracheal tube (Combitube): confirmation of placement is essential

See Bag-Mask Ventilation on page 10-24.

Considerations / Notes	
Cricoid Pressure	• Is not routinely recommended • May help prevent gastric inflation. • Use only if victim is deeply unconscious (no cough or gag reflex). • Usually requires third rescuer
Regurgitation	• If patient vomits, turn to side, wipe out mouth, return to supine, and continue CPR
Capnography/ Capnometry	• Continuous quantitative waveform capnography is recommended for intubated patients through the peri-arrest period for: • Confirming tracheal tube placement • Monitoring CPR quality and therapy • Detecting ROSC based upon end-tidal carbon dioxide ($PetCO_2$) values • If $PetCO_2$ <10 mm Hg, attempt to improve CPR quality • An abrupt and sustained rise in $PetCO_2$ may be observed just before clinical identification of ROSC, so use of $PetCO_2$ monitoring may reduce the need to interrupt chest compressions for a pulse check. • Falling cardiac output or rearrest in the patient with ROSC causes a decrease in $PetCO_2$.

Monitoring	
Pulses	• Take < 10 sec to palpate for pulse; resume compressions immediately in unable to feel. • Carotid pulsations during CPR do not indicate the efficacy of coronary, myocardial or cerebral perfusion. Femoral pulsations may indicate venous rather than arterial flow • If A-line monitor: maximize BP dia (ideally ≥30 – 10 = 20 mmHg)
Oximetry	• During arrest, SpO_2 is a poor indicator • Upon ROSC, use $SpO2$ to titrate inspired Oxygen (when equipment available) - maintain an $SaO2$ ≥ 94%, but < 100% to limit the risk of hyperoxemia. • $ScvO_2$: Indicator of CO and O_2 delivery during CPR. If CVP line in place, can you monitor CPR effectiveness (should be > 30%) and detect ROSC without interrupting chest compressions to check rhythm and pulse.
ABG's	Not a reliable indicator of the severity of tissue hypoxemia, hypercarbia (ie., ventilation), or tissue acidosis during arrest
$ETCO_2$	• Safe and effective indicator of CO (+ may be ROSC) during CPR • If ventilation is reasonably constant: $\Delta CO2 \approx \Delta CO$ • An abrupt sustained increase in $PETCO_2$ during CPR is an indicator of ROSC. • A transient rise in $PETCO_2$ after sodium bicarbonate therapy is expected and should not be misinterpreted as an improvement in quality of CPR or a sign of ROSC. • Persistently low $PETCO_2$ values (< 10 mm Hg) during CPR in intubated pts suggest that ROSC is unlikely. • Monitoring $PETCO_2$ trends during CPR has the potential to guide individual optimization of compression depth and rate and to detect fatigue in the provider performing compressions. • After CPR – use to guide ventil. (along w/ ABG) + ET tube position

Cardiac Arrest in Special Situations

See Oakes' www.RespiratoryUpdate.com for a quick reference synopsis of Cardiopulmonary Resuscitation and Emergency Cardiovascular Care in the following Special Situations, to include BLS and ACLS Modifications:

- Asthma
- Anaphylaxis
- Avalanche Victims
- Cardiac Tamponade
- Drowning
- During Percutaneous Coronary Intervention
- Electric Shock and Lightning Strikes
- Following Cardiac Surgery
- Hypothermia
- Life-Threatening Electrolyte Disturbances
- Morbidly Obese
- Pregnancy
- Pulmonary Embolism
- Toxic Ingestions (including CO Poisoning)
- Trauma

POST-RESUSCITATION SUPPORT

Recommendations
1. Optimize cardiopulmonary function and vital organ perfusion after ROSC
2. Transport/transfer to an appropriate hospital or critical care unit with a comprehensive post–cardiac arrest treatment system of care
3. Identify and treat ACS and other reversible causes

H's	T's
Hypoxia	Toxins
Hypovolemia	Trauma
Hyperthermia	Thrombosis
Hypoglycemia	Tamponade (cardiac)
Hypo/hyperkalemia	Tension pneumothorax
Hydrogen ion (acidosis)	Treat consequences (hypoxia, ischemia, reperfusion)

4. Control temperature to optimize neurologic recovery
5. Anticipate, treat, and prevent multiple organ dysfunction. This includes avoiding excessive ventilation and hyperoxia

Withdrawal of Life Support

Ethically permissible when:
- No motor response at 24 hrs
- No motor response at 72 hrs
- Absent corneal reflex at 24 hrs
- Absent pupillary response at 24 hrs
- Absent withdrawal response to pain at 24 hrs

Ventilation	
Capnography	• Confirm secure airway and titrate ventilation • ET Tube when possible for comatose patients • $PETCO_2 \approx 35–40$ mm Hg • $PaCO_2 \approx 40–45$ mm Hg
CXR	Confirm secure airway and detect causes or complications of arrest: pneumonitis, pneumonia, pulmonary edema

Pulse Oximetry/ ABG	• Maintain adequate oxygenation and minimize FIO_2
	  • $SpO_2 \geq 94\%$
	  • $PaO_2 \approx 100$ mmHg
	• Reduce FIO_2 as tolerated
	• PaO_2/FIO_2 ratio to follow acute lung injury

Mechanical Ventilation	• Minimize acute lung injury, potential oxygen toxicity
	• Tidal Volume 6–8 mL/kg
	• Titrate minute ventilation to
	  • $PETCO_2 \approx 35–40$ mm Hg
	  • $PaCO_2 \approx 40–45$ mm Hg
	• Avoid hyperventilation *
	• Reduce FiO_2 as tolerated to keep SpO_2 or $SaO2 \geq 94\%$

* Achieve normocarbia – avoid hyperventilation
After ROSC, there is commonly a brief period (10-30 min) of cerebral hyperemia, followed by a prolonged period of hyperemia.
Potential detrimental effects of hyperventilation:

$\uparrow$ PIT $\rightarrow$ $\downarrow$CO $\rightarrow$ $\downarrow$cerebral blood flow $\rightarrow$ $\uparrow$ ischemia

$\downarrow$PCO2 $\rightarrow$ cerebral vasoconstriction $\rightarrow$ $\downarrow$cerebral blood flow $\rightarrow$ $\uparrow$ ischemia

$\uparrow$ Paw and/or $\uparrow$ auto-PEEP $\rightarrow$ $\uparrow$ intracranial pressure, $\rightarrow$ $\downarrow$cerebral blood flow $\rightarrow$ $\uparrow$ ischemia

Hemodynamics	
Freq BP Monitoring/ A-Line	• Maintain perfusion and prevent recurrent hypotension • Mean Arterial Pressure ≥65 mm Hg or systolic blood pressure ≥ 90 mm Hg
Treat Hypotension	Maintain perfusion; Fluid bolus if tolerated Dopamine 5–10 mcg/kg per min Norepinephrine 0.1–0.5 mcg/kg per min Epinephrine 0.1–0.5 mcg/kg per min

Cardiovascular
Continuous Cardiac Monitoring
12-lead ECG/Troponin, Echocardiogram
Treat Myocardial Stunning and Acute Coronary Syndrome

Neurological	
Serial Neuro Exam	• Define coma, brain injury, and prognosis • Response to verbal commands or physical stimulation • Pupillary light and coronary reflex, spont eye movement • Gag, cough, spontaneous breaths
EEG Monitoring if Coma	• Exclude seizures • Anticonvulsants if seizing
Sedation/ Muscle Relaxation	• To control shivering, agitation, or ventilator dyssynchrony as needed

Metabolic	
Serial Lactate	• Confirm adequate perfusion
Serum Potassium	• Avoid hypokalemia which promotes arrhythmias • Replace to maintain K > 3.5 mEq/L

Urine Output, Serum Creatinine
Serum Glucose
Avoid Hypotonic Fluid

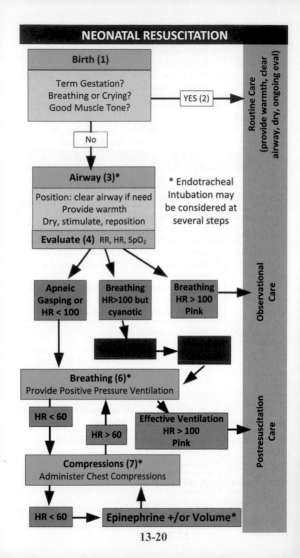

NEONATAL RESUSCITATION

Birth (1)

Term Gestation?
Breathing or Crying?
Good Muscle Tone?

→ YES (2) →

Routine Care (provide warmth, clear airway, dry, ongoing eval)

No ↓

Airway (3)*

Position: clear airway if need
Provide warmth
Dry, stimulate, reposition

Evaluate (4) RR, HR, SpO₂

* Endotracheal Intubation may be considered at several steps

Apneic Gasping or HR < 100

Breathing HR>100 but cyanotic

Breathing HR > 100 Pink →

Observational Care

Breathing (6)*
Provide Positive Pressure Ventilation

HR < 60

HR > 60

Effective Ventilation HR > 100 Pink →

Compressions (7)*
Administer Chest Compressions

HR < 60 → **Epinephrine +/or Volume***

Postresuscitation Care

13-20

FOOTNOTES

(1) Guidelines apply to neonates at birth and first few months.
   CPR Indications:
   All conditions assoc. with high rate of survival and acceptable morbidity (includes ≥ 25 wk gestation [unless fetal compromise] and most congenital malformations).
   CPR Not Indicated:
   Almost certain death and high morbidity expected (includes < 23 wk or < 400 g, anencephaly, and chromosomal abnormalities).
   CPR Questionable:
   Uncertain prognosis, survival borderline, and high morbidity and burden – support parental desires
   Note: The majority of newborns who will need resuscitation can be identified before birth. At least one person who can perform a complete resuscitation should be at every delivery. Additional skilled personnel should be recruited if resuscitation is anticipated. Special preparations are required for preterm delivery (< 37 wk). Further info available at www.aap.org/NRP.

(2) Routine Care: Do not separate baby from mother

(3) **AIRWAY**
   Initial steps of resuscitation:
   Place baby under radiant heat
   LBW (< 1500 g) – use additional warming techniques (e.g., plastic wrapping).
   Monitor temperature closely; avoid hyperthermia
   Position head in "sniffing" position to open airway
   Clear airway with bulb syringe or suction catheter only if baby has airway obstruction or requires PPV.
   Dry baby and stimulate breathing

   Meconium staining:
   Routine intrapartum suctioning no longer advised
   Vigorous infant (HR > 100, strong respiratory effort, good muscle tone) – do not perform ET suctioning
   Not vigorous – perform ET suctioning immediately after birth

(4) Evaluate – simultaneous assessment of all 3 (RR, HR, SpO$_2$ [in < 30 sec])
   HR is a good indicator of improvement or deterioration
   Reassess all 3 (RR, HR, SpO$_2$) every 30 sec

(5) *Oxygen*

Indication: SpO$_2$ level

Dosage:

Term Babies: Begin resuscitation with air

O2 administration should be guided by SpO2 (pulse ox on upper right extremity; i.e. wrist or palm)

Notes:

Assess simultaneously: HR, RR, SpO2

If no O2 available, give PPV with room air

Guide administration with pulse oximetry

Avoid excessive O2 in the premature infant

Healthy term babies may take > 10 min to reach preductal O2 Sat > 95% and 1 hr to reach postductal O2 Sat > 95%.

Pallor or mottling may be a sign of ↓ CO, severe anemia, hypovolemia, hypothermia, or acidosis.

Targeted Preductal SpO2 after birth:

1 min	60-65%
2 min	65-70%
3 min	70-75%
4 min	75-80%
10 min	85-95%

(6) BREATHING (PPV)

Initial Parameters

Rate: 40 – 60 breaths/min (to achieve/maintain HR > 100)
(Assess chest wall movement if HR does not improve)

PIP: 30 – 40 cm H2O

(Individualize to achieve ↑ HR and/or chest movement)

If monitored, 20 cmH2O may be effective

If not monitored, use minimum inflation required to achieve ↑ HR.

Preterm infants

PIP: 20 to 25 cm H2O

Adequate for most

↑ if no prompt ↑ in HR or chest movement

Avoid excessive chest wall movement.

Monitor PIP if possible

PEEP or CPAP may be beneficial

Endotracheal intubation
INDICATIONS

Bag/mask ineffective or prolonged	Administration of medications
When chest compressions are performed	CDH or extremely low birthweight (< 1000 g)
Tracheal suctioning for meconium	

Check tube position:
Best indicator is ↑ HR
Chest movement (present or absent)
Condensation during exhalation
Confirm visually during intubation
Confirm with exhale CO_2 detector after intubation

(7) CHEST COMPRESSIONS
Ensure assisted ventilation is being delivered optimally before starting chest compressions.
Ventilation/compressions are synchronized (pause compressions)

Method:	Depth: 1/3 of chest A-P dia
2 thumb-encircling technique – recommended	I:E: slightly > 1:1
2 finger technique – optional	Rate: 90 compressions/min
	Ratio: 3:1
Position: lower 1/3 of sternum	(90 compressions + 30 breaths)
	(120 events/min; ½ sec each)
	if known cardiac, consider 15:2
	2 rescuer
	Continue until HR ≥ 60/min

Guidelines for Witholding and Discontinuing Resuscitation	
Witholding	When congential anomalies, birth weight, and gestation are associated with high morbidity and almost certain early death, resuscitation is not indicated.
Discontinuation	• Discontinuation is justified after 10 min of continuous and adequate resuscitation if the HR remains undetectable for 10 min. • Consideration factors include: presumed etiology, gestation, presence or absence of complications, potential role of therapeutic hypothermia, and the parents' previously expressed feelings.

ADDITIONAL RESOURCES

See Oakes' **RespiratoryUpdate.com** for further information and explanations of CPR, including direct links to:

Evidence-Based Guidelines
- 2010 American Heart Association Guidelines for Cardiopulmonary Resuscitation and Emergency Cardiovascular Care Science
- Highlights of the 2010 American Heart Association Guidelines for CPR and ECC
- ACLS Algorithm Flowcharts, October 2010 Guidelines

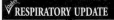

RESPIRATORY UPDATE

THE Virtual Critical Care Library

A Appendix

Symbols

Basic Units of Measure

cmH₂0	centimeters of water pressure		
°C	degrees of temperature in centigrade	sec	seconds
ft	foot	m	meters
gm%	gram percent (number of grams per 100 grams of total weight)	vol%	volume percent (number of mL of a substance per 100 mL of total volume)
in.	inch	beats/min(bpm)	heart beats per minute
kcal	kilocalorie	breaths/min	breaths per minute
kg	kilograms	L/min	liters per minute
kPa	SI unit for pressure*	L/sec	liters per second
l or L	liters	mEq/L	milliequivalents per liter
L/kPa	SI unti for compliance*	mg/mL	milligrams per milliliter
mL	milliliters	mL/min	milliliters per minute
min	minutes	mL/kg	milliliters per kilogram
mM	millimole	SI	standard international unit*
mmHg	millimeters of mercury pressure		

SI equivalents: kPa=mmHg x 0.133   L/kPa=L/cmH20 x 10.2   kPa=cmH20 x 0.098

Basic Gas Phase Symbols

Primary Symbols

D	diffusion	R	respiratory exchange ratio
F	fractional concentration of a gas	V	volume of gas
P	partial pressure of a gas	$\dot{V}$	flow of gas (volume/time)
$\overline{P}$	mean pressure of a gas		

Qualifying Subscripts

anat	anatomic	E	expired	BTPS	body conditions: body temperature and ambient pressure, saturated with water vapor at these conditions
aw	airway	I	inspired		
dyn	dynamic	L	lung		
eso	esophagus	S	static	ATPD	ambient temp and press, dry
f	frequency	T	tidal	ATPS	ambient temperature and pressure, saturated with water vapor at these conditions
phy	physiologic	CO2	carbon dioxide		
pl	pleural	O2	oxygen		
stat	static	N2	nitrogen	STPD	standard conditions: temperature 0°C, pressure 760 torr, and dry (0 torr water vapor)
t	time	H20	water		
A(alv)	alveolar				
B	barometric				
D	deadspace				

Basic Blood Phase Symbols

Primary Symbols		Qualifying Subscripts	
Q	volume of blood	a	arterial
$\dot{Q}$	blood flow (cardiac output), L/min	c	capillary
C	concentration (content in the blood phase)	c	pulmonary end - capillary
		s	shunt
S	saturation in the blood phase	v	venous
		$\overline{v}$	mixed venous

A-2

Abbreviations

Abbrev.	Definition	Abbrev.	Definition	Abbrev.	Definition	Abbrev.	Definition
AARC	American Association of Respiratory Care	bpm	Beats or breaths/minute	COPD	Chronic obstructive pulmonary disease	ECG	Electrocardiogram
ABG	Arterial blood gas	BPsys	Systolic blood pressure	CPAP	Continuous positive airway pressure	ECMO	Extracorporeal membrane oxygenation
A/C	Assist/control	B-P	Broncho-pleural	CPG	Clinical Practice Guideline	EDV	End diastolic volume
ACCP	American College of Chest Physicians	BSA	Body surface area	CPP	Cerebral or coronary perfusion pressure	EEP	End expiratory pressure
ACLS	Advanced Cardiac Life Support	CABG	Coronary artery bypass graph	CPR	Cardio-pulmonary resuscitation	EGTA	Esophageal-gastric tube airway
ADH	Anti-diuretic hormone	CaO_2	Arterial oxygen content	CPT	Chest physical therapy	EKG	Electrocardiogram
A-fib	Atrial fibrillation	$Ca\text{-}\overline{V}O_2$	Arterial –mixed venous O_2 content difference	CSF	Cerebral spinal fluid	EPAP	Expiratory positive airway pressure
AG	Anion gap	CB	Chronic Bronchitis	Cstat	Static compliance	ERV	Expiratory reserve volume
AHA	American Heart Assoc	CC	Closing capacity	Ctubing	Compliance of the tubing	et	End-tidal
ALI	Acute lung injury	Ccw	Chest wall compliance	CV	Cardiovascular	ET	Endotracheal
AMI	Acute Myocardial infarct	CHD	Congenital heart disease	CVA	Cerebrovascular accident	ETS	Endotracheal suction
A-P	Anterior-Posterior	CHF	Congestive heart failure	CvO_2	Venous oxygen content	EIA	Exercise induced asthma
ARDS	Acute respiratory distress syndrome	Cdyn	Dynamic compliance	CVP	Central venous pressure	f	Frequency (ventilator rate)
ARF	Acute respiratory failure	CF	Conversion factor/Cystic Fibrosis	CXR	Chest x-ray	FDO_2	Fraction of delivered O_2
ASD	Atrial septal defect	CI	Cardiac index	D	Deadspace or diffusion	$FECO_2$	Fractional concentration of expired CO_2
AV	Atrio-ventricular	CL	Compliance of the lung	DKA	Diabetic ketoacidosis	FEF	Forced expiratory flow
a-v	arterio-venous	CLT	Compliance of the lung and thorax	DLCO	Diffusion capacity for CO	FEV	Forced expiratory volume
BE/BD	Base excess/deficit	cm H_2O	Centimeters of water	DO_2	Oxygen delivery	FICO	Fraction of inspired CO
BiPAP	Bi-level positive airway pressure	CMV	Cytomegaly virus	DOE	Dyspnea on exertion	FIF	Forced inspiratory flow
BLS	Basic Life Support	CNS	Central nervous system	DPG,2,3	2,3 diphosphglycerate	FIO_2	Fraction of inspired oxygen
BP	Blood pressure	CO	Cardiac output	DPI	Dry powder inhaler	FIVC	Forced inspiratory vital capacity
BPdia	Diastolic blood pressure	CO	Carbon monoxide	E	Expiration	Fr	French
		CO_2	Carbon dioxide	ECC	Emergency cardiac care		

FRC	Functional residual capacity
F-T	Flow-time
FVC	Forced vital capacity
Gaw	Airway conductance
GI	Gastrointestinal
H+	Hydrogen ion
HbO2	Oxyhemoglobin
HCH	Hygroscopic condenser humidifier
HCO3	Bicarbonate
Hct	Hematocrit
HFV	High frequency ventilation
Hgb	Hemoglobin
HME	Heat moisture exchanger
HR	Heart rate or heated reservoir
I	Inspiration
IC	Inspiratory capacity
ICP	Intracranial pressure
ID	Internal diameter
I:E	Inspiratory/expiratory ratio
IPAP	Inspiratory positive airway pressure
IMV	Intermittent mandatory ventilation
IO	Intraosseous
I+O	Intake & output
IPPB	Intermittent positive pressure breathing
IRV	Inspiratory reserve volume or Inverse ratio ventilation
IS	Incentive spirometry
IV	Intravenous
J	Joule
JVD	Jugular vein distention
kg	Kilogram
LA	Left atrium
LAP	Left atrial pressure
LDH	Lactic dehydrogenase
LOC	Level of consciousness
L-R	Left to right
LV	Left ventricle
LHF	Left heart failure
LVF	Left ventricular failure
LVH	Left ventricular hypertrophy
LVEDP	Left ventricular end diastolic pressure
LVEDV	Left ventricular end diastolic volume
LVESP	Left ventricular end systolic pressure
LVESV	Left ventricular end systolic volume
LVSW	Left ventricular stroke work
LVSWI	Left ventricular stroke work index
MAP	Mean arterial pressure
MBC	Maximum breathing capacity
MDI	Metered dose inhaler
MDO2	Myocardial oxygen delivery
MEF	Maximal expiratory pressure
MEFV	Maximal expiratory flow volume
MI	Myocardial infarction
MIF	See PImax
MIP	See PImax
mm Hg	millimeters of mercury
MvO2	Myocardial O2 consumption
MV	Mechanical ventilation
MVV	Maximum voluntary ventilation
NG	Nasogastric
NIF	See PImax
N-M	Neuromuscular
NO	Nitric oxide
NPPV	Noninvasive positive pressure ventilation
NSS	Normal saline solution
NTS	Nasotracheal suction
O2	Oxygen
O2ER	Oxygen extraction ratio
O2 Sat	Oxygen saturation
P	Pressure
PA	Pulmonary artery or posterior-anterior
PA-aO2	Alveolar-arterial oxygen partial pressure difference
PaCO2	Partial pressure of arterial carbon dioxide
PACO2	Partial pressure of alveolar carbon dioxide
PAC	Premature atrial contraction
P-ACV	Pressure-assist/control ventilation
PAPD	Pulmonary artery diastolic pressure
PAEPD	Pulmonary artery end-diastolic pressure
Palv	Alveolar pressure
PAMP	Pulmonary artery mean pressure
PaO2	Partial pressure of arterial oxygen
PAO2	Partial pressure of alveolar oxygen
PAOP	Pulmonary artery occlusion pressure
PAP	Pulmonary artery pressure
PASP	Pulmonary artery systolic pressure
PAT	Premature atrial tachycardia
Paw	Airway pressure
Paw‾	Mean airway pressure
Pawo	Pressure at airway opening

PAWP	Pulmonary artery wedge pressure
PB	Barometric pressure
PBW	Predicted body weight
PCWP	Pulmonary capillary wedge pressure
Pcyl	Pressure in a cylinder
PDT	Postural drainage therapy
PEA	Pulseless electrical activity
PECO2	Partial pressure of expired CO2
PetCO2	Partial pressure of end-expired CO2
PEEP	Positive end-expiratory pressure
PEF	Peak expiratory flow
PEP	Positive expiratory pressure
PFT	Pulmonary function test
pH	Negative log of hydrogen ion concentration
pHa	pH of arterial blood
pHv	pH of venous blood
PIF	Peak inspiratory flow
PImax	Maximal inspiratory pressure
PIO2	Partial pressure of inspired O2
PIP	Peak inspiratory pressure
PIT	Intrathoracic pressure
PIV	Intravascular pressure
PMI	Point of maximal impulse
PNC	Premature nodal contraction
PND	Paroxysmal nocturnal dyspnea
PP	Pulse pressure
PPE	Personal Protective Equipment
Ppl	Intrapleural pressure
Ppeak	Peak inspiratory pressure
Pplat	Inspiratory plateau pressure
PPV	Positive pressure ventilation
PSTV	Paroxysmal supra-ventricular tachycardia
PT	Prothrombin time
PtcO2	Transcutaneous partial pressure of oxygen
PTL	Pharyngo-tracheal lumen airway
Ptm	Transmural pressure
PTT	Partial prothrombin time
PV	Pressure ventilation
PVC	Premature ventricular contraction
PVD	Peripheral vascular disease
PYO2	Partial pressure of oxygen in mixed venous blood
PVR	Pulmonary vascular resistance
PVRI	Pulmonary vascular resistance index
P50	Pressure at 50% saturation
Q	Perfusion
Qc pul	Pulmonary capillary blood volume
Qpul	Pulmonary perfusion
Qs	Shunt
Qs anat	Anatomical shunt
Qs cap	Capillary shunt
Qs/Qt	Physiological shunt
QT	Total perfusion
R(RR)	Respiratory exchange ratio
Raw	Airway resistance
RA	Right atrium
RHF	Right heart failure
RAP	Right atrial pressure
RBC	Red blood cell
RFF	Ratio flow factor
RH	Right heart
RHF	Right heart failure
R-L	Right to left
ROSC	Return of spontaneous circulation
R pul	Pulmonary resistance
RQ	Respiratory quotient
RR	Spontaneous respiratory rate
RV	Right ventricle
RVEDP	Right ventricle end-diastolic pressure
RVEDV	Right ventricular end diastolic volume
RVESP	Right ventricular end systolic pressure
RVESV	Right ventricular end systolic volume
RVF	Right ventricular failure
RVSW	Right ventricular stroke work
RVSWI	Right ventricular stroke work index
SA	Sino-atrial
SaO2	Saturation of arterial oxygen
Sat	Saturation
SBN2	Single breath nitrogen washout
SCCM	Society of Critical Care Medicine
SMI	Sustained maximal inspiration
SOB	Shortness of breath
SPAG	Small particle aerosol generator
SpO2	Saturation of arterial oxygen

A-6

Metric Measurements

Linear		Weight		Volume	
kilometer (km)	m × 10³	kilogram (kg)	g × 10³	kiloliter	1 × 10³
decameter	m × 10	decagram	g × 10	decaliter	1 × 10
meter (m)		gram (g)		liter (L)	
decimeter	m × 10⁻¹	decigram	g × 10⁻¹	deciliter (dL)	1 × 10⁻¹
centimeter (cm)	m × 10⁻²	centigram	g × 10⁻²	centiliter	1 × 10⁻²
millimeter (mm)	m × 10⁻³	milligram (mg)	g × 10⁻³	milliliter (mL)	1 × 10⁻³
micrometer (μ or μm)	m × 10⁻⁶	microgram (μg)	g × 10⁻⁶	microliter (μL)	1 × 10⁻⁶

U.S. Customary and Metric Equivalents

Linear		Weight		Volume	
1 inch	2.54 cm	1 ounce (oz)	28.35g	1 ounce (fl)	29.57 mL
1 foot	.0348 m	1 pound	454 g	1 quart	0.9463 L
1 mile	1.609 km	1 gram	0.0352 oz	1 gallon	3.785 L
1 micron	3.937 x 10⁻⁵ in	1 kilogram	2.2 lb	cubic inch	16.39 mL
1 centimeter	0.3937 in			cubic foot	28.32 L
1 meter	39.37 in			1 liter	1.057 qt
1 kilometer	0.6214 mile				61.02 in³
					0.03532 ft³

Conversion Tables					
Temperature				**Length**	
°C = (°F-32) x 5/9		°F = (°C x 9/5) + 32		1 inch = 2.54 cm	
°F	°C	°C	°F	inch	cm
0	-17.7	0	32	1	2.5
95	35.0	35.0	95.0	2	5.1
96	35.5	35.5	95.9	4	10.2
97	36.1	36.0	96.8	6	15.2
98	36.6	36.5	97.7	8	20.3
99	37.2	37.0	98.6	12	30.5
100	37.7	37.5	99.5	18	46
101	38.3	38.0	100.4	24	61
102	38.8	38.5	101.3	30	76
103	39.4	39.0	102.2	36	91
104	40.0	39.5	103.1	42	107
105	40.5	40.0	104.0	48	122
106	41.1	40.5	104.9	54	137
107	41.6	41.0	105.8	60	152
108	42.2	41.5	106.6	66	168
109	42.7	42.0	107.6	72	183
110	43.3	100.0	212.0	78	198

Weight				Pressure	
1 lb = 0.454 kg		1 kg = 2.2 lb		1.36cmH20 = 1 mmHg 1 cmH20 = 0.098 kPa 1 cmH20 = 0.735 mmHg 1 mmHg = 0.133 kPa	
lb	kg	kg	lb	cmH20	mmHg
1	0.5	1	2.2	6.8	5
2	0.9	2	4.4	13.6	10
4	1.8	3	6.6	20.4	15
6	2.7	4	8.8	27.2	20
8	3.6	5	11.0	33.9	25
10	4.5	6	13.2	40.7	30
20	9.1	8	17.6	47.5	35
30	13.6	10	22	54.3	40
40	18.3	20	44	61.1	45
50	22.7	30	66	1 PSIG	70.31 cmH20
60	27.3	40	88	1	760 mmHg
70	31.8	50	110	atmosphere	14.7 psi
80	36.4	60	132		0 psi (gauge)
90	40.9	70	154		1034 cmH20
100	45.4	80	176		
150	69.2	90	198		
200	90.8	100	220		

Infection Control Guidelines

CDC Standard Precautions	
Applies to:	1) All patients (regardless of diagnosis or infection status).
	2) Blood, all body fluids, secretions, excretions (except sweat), non-intact skin, and mucous membranes.
Handwashing	Wash hands after; touching blood, body fluids, secretions, excretions, or contaminated items (even if wearing gloves); immediately after removing gloves; between patient contacts; between tasks/procedures on different body sites of the same patient; and when otherwise indicated. Use plain soap for routine handwashing and antimicrobial soap or waterless antiseptic for specific instances.
Gloves	Wear clean gloves when touching blood, body fluids, secretions, excretions, contaminated items, mucous membranes, and nonintact skin. Change gloves between tasks/procedures on same patient after contact within the infectious material. Remove gloves promptly after use, before touching noncontaminated items or surfaces, and before going to another patient. Wash hands immediately after removing gloves.
Gowns	Wear a clean gown to protect skin and clothing from splashes or sprays of blood, body fluids, secretions, or excretions. Remove soiled gown as promptly as possible and wash hands.
Patient Care Equipment	Handle used equipment soiled with blood, body fluids, secretions, and excretions in a manner that prevents skin and mucous membrane exposure, contamination of clothing, and transfer of microorganisms to other patients and/or environments. Do not use reusable equipment for another patient unless cleaned/reprocessed appropriately. Properly discard single-use items.
Occupational Health and Blood-borne Pathogens	Use extreme caution when handling, cleaning, or disposing of needles, scalpels, and other sharp instruments or devices. Never recap, use both hands, or point towards the body any used needles; rather, use either a one-handed "scoop" technique or a mechanical device. Do not bend, break, manipulate, or remove used needles from disposable syringes by hand. Place used disposable syringes and needles, scalpel blades, and other sharp items in appropriate puncture-resistant containers; place reusable syringes and needles in a puncture-resistant container to be reprocessed. Use mouthpieces, resuscitation bags, or other ventilation devices as an alternative to mouth to mouth resuscitation.
Patient Placement	Use a private room for patients who contaminate the environment or who do not/cannot assist in maintaining appropriate hygiene or environmental control. Consult with infection control if a private room is not available.
Mask, Eye Protection, Face Shield:	Wear to protect eyes, nose, and mouth from splashes/sprays of blood,/body fluids,/secretions/excretions.

A-9

Transmission-Based Precautions

Additional precautions beyond Standard Precautions.

Applies to: Patients with known or suspected infections (or colonized) with pathogens that can be transmitted by airborne, droplet, or contact.

Airborne Precautions (Small particle airborne droplet nuclei)	**Patient Placement:** Private negative-pressure room with 6 to12 air changes/hr, plus either safe external air discharge or HEPA filtration. Cohorting acceptable or consult with infection control. Keep room door closed and patient in room. **Patient Transport:** Essential purposes only. Have patient wear a surgical mask. **Respiratory Protection:** Wear N95 respirator when entering room of patient with known/suspected infectious pulmonary TB. Persons immune to measles (rubeola) or varice la (chickenpox) need not wear respiratory protection. If possible, persons not immune to measles or varicella should not enter the room, or wear respiratory protection.
Droplet Precautions (Large droplets)	**Patient Placement:** Private room, cohorting acceptable, or separate patient from others (patients and visitors) by > 3 feet. **Patient Transport:** Essential purposes only. Have patient wear a surgical mask. **Mask:** Wear a surgical mask within 3 ft. of patient (or upon entering room).
Contact Precautions (Hand or skin-to-skin contact)	**Patient Placement:** Private room, cohorting acceptable, or consult with infection control. **Patient Transport:** Essential purposes only. If must be transported, minimize risk of disease transmission. **Gloves and Handwashing:** Wear clean gloves upon entering room. Change gloves after contact with infectious material. Remove gloves before leaving patient's environment and wash hands immediately with antimicrobial agent or waterless antiseptic. Then do not touch any potentially contaminated surface or item. **Gown:** Wear clean gown upon entering room: if anticipate patient, surface, or item contact; if patient incontinent, has diarrhea, ileostomy, colostomy, or wound drainage not contained by a dressing. Remove gown before leaving room, then do not contact any potentially contaminated surface. **Patient Care Equipment:** Dedicate use of noncritical equipment to single patient or cohort. If shared, ensure adequately cleaned and disinfected before next patient use.

* Guideline for Isolation Precautions: Preventing Transmission of Infectious Agents in Healthcare Settings 2007. http://www.cdc.gov/ncidod/dhqp/pdf/guidelines/Isolation2007.pdf

A-10

Index